Complementary and Integrative Therapies for Psychiatric Disorders

Editors

PHILIP R. MUSKIN
PATRICIA L. GERBARG
RICHARD P. BROWN

PSYCHIATRIC CLINICS OF NORTH AMERICA

www.psych.theclinics.com

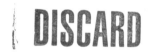

March 2013 • Volume 36 • Number 1

ELSEVIER

1600 John F. Kennedy Boulevard • Suite 1800 • Philadelphia, Pennsylvania, 19103-2899

http://www.theclinics.com

PSYCHIATRIC CLINICS OF NORTH AMERICA Volume 36, Number 1
March 2013 ISSN 0193-953X, ISBN-13: 978-1-4557-7147-9

Editor: Joanne Husovski
Developmental Editor: Donald Mumford

Psychiatric Clinics of North America (ISSN 0193-953X) is published quarterly by Elsevier Inc., 360 Park Avenue South, New York, NY 10010-1710. Months of issue are March, June, September, and December. Business and Editorial Offices: 1600 John F. Kennedy Blvd., Suite 1800, Philadelphia, PA 19103-2899. Periodicals postage paid at New York, NY and additional mailing offices. Subscription prices are $286.00 per year (US individuals), $524.00 per year (US institutions), $141.00 per year (US students/residents), $347.00 per year (Canadian individuals), $651.00 per year (Canadian Institutions), $431.00 per year (foreign individuals), $651.00 per year (foreign institutions), and $210.00 per year (international & Canadian students/residents). Foreign air speed delivery is included in all Clinics' subscription prices. All prices are subject to change without notice. **POSTMASTER:** Send address changes to Psychiatric Clinics of North America, Elsevier Health Sciences Division, Subscription Customer Service, 3251 Riverport Lane, Maryland Heights, MO 63043. Customer Service: 1-800-654-2452 (US). From outside the United States, call 1-314-447-8871. Fax: 1-314-447-8029. E-mail: journalscustomerservice-usa@elsevier.com (for print support) and journalsonlinesupport-usa@elsevier.com (for online support).

Reprints. For copies of 100 or more, of articles in this publication, please contact the Commercial Reprints Department, Elsevier Inc., 360 Park Avenue South, New York, New York 10010-1710. Tel.: (212) 633-3813, Fax: (212) 462-1935, E-mail: reprints@elsevier.com.

Psychiatric Clinics of North America is covered in MEDLINE/PubMed (Index Medicus), Current Contents/Social and Behavioral Sciences, Social Science Citation Index, Embase/Excerpta Medica, and PsycINFO.

Printed in the United States of America.

Contributors

EDITORS

PHILIP R. MUSKIN, MD
Professor of Clinical Psychiatry, Columbia University College of Physicians and Surgeons, Chief, Consultation-Liaison Psychiatry, NY-Presbyterian Hospital/Columbia Campus, New York, New York

PATRICIA L. GERBARG, MD
Assistant Professor of Clinical Psychiatry, Department of Psychiatry, New York Medical College, Valhalla, New York

RICHARD P. BROWN, MD
Associate Professor of Clinical Psychiatry, Department of Psychiatry, Columbia University College of Physicians and Surgeons, New York, New York

AUTHORS

RYAN ABBOTT, MD, JD, MTOM
Associate Professor of Law at Southwestern Law School, Los Angeles, California

SHAHIN AKHONDZADEH, PhD, FBPharmacolS
Professor of Clinical Neuroscience, Psychiatric Research Center, Roozbeh Hospital, Tehran University of Medical Sciences, Tehran, Iran

MARY R. BAILEY, MA
Clinical Research Assistant, Neuropsychology, Cognitive Neuroscience, and Clinical Outcomes Laboratory, Department of Psychology, William Paterson University, Wayne, New Jersey

TEODORO BOTTIGLIERI, PhD
Principal Investigator, Adjunct Professor of Biomedical Sciences, Institute of Metabolic Disease, Baylor Research Institute, Baylor University, Dallas, Texas

KELLY BROGAN, MD, ABIHM
Clinical Instructor, NYU/Bellevue Hospital Center, New York, New York

RICHARD P. BROWN, MD
Associate Professor of Clinical Psychiatry, Department of Psychiatry, Columbia University College of Physicians and Surgeons, New York, New York

BRUCE J. DIAMOND, PhD
Professor, Graduate Program Director, Director of Neuropsychology, Cognitive Neuroscience, and Clinical Outcomes Laboratory, Department of Psychology, William Paterson University, Wayne, New Jersey

LESTER G. FEHMI, PhD
Clinical Director, Princeton Biofeedback Centre, Princeton, New Jersey

MARLENE P. FREEMAN, MD
Department of Psychiatry, Massachusetts General Hospital, Harvard Medical School; Director of Clinical Services, Perinatal and Reproductive Psychiatry Program, Harvard Medical School, Boston, Massachusetts

PATRICIA L. GERBARG, MD
Assistant Professor of Clinical Psychiatry, Department of Psychiatry, New York Medical College, Valhalla, New York

DANIEL L. KIRSCH, PhD
President, The American Institute of Stress, Fort Worth, Texas

STEPHEN LARSEN, PhD
LMHC, Licensed Mental Health Counselor, NY, BCN, Board Certified in Neurofeedback (BCIA), Stone Mountain Center, New Paltz; Psychology Professor Emeritus, SUNY, Ulster, Stone Ridge, New York

HELEN LAVRETSKY, MD, MS
Professor of Psychiatry, Department of Psychiatry and Biobehavioral Sciences, Semel Institute for Neuroscience and Human Behavior, David Geffen School of Medicine at UCLA, Los Angeles, California

WILLIAM R. MARCHAND, MD
Psychiatrist, George E. Wahlen Veterans Administration Medical Center; Associate Professor (Clinical), Department of Psychiatry, University of Utah, Salt Lake City, Utah

DAVID MISCHOULON, MD, PhD
Director of Research, Depression Clinical and Research Program, Massachusetts General Hospital, Associate Professor of Psychiatry, Harvard Medical School; Department of Psychiatry, Massachusetts General Hospital, Harvard Medical School, Boston, Massachusetts

AMIRHOSSEIN MODABBERNIA, MD
Psychiatry Research Fellow, Psychiatric Research Center, Roozbeh Hospital, Tehran University of Medical Sciences, Tehran, Iran

FRED MUENCH, PhD
Assistant Professor of Psychology, Columbia University College of Physicians and Surgeons, New York, New York

FRANCINE NICHOLS, RN, PhD
Professor (retired), Georgetown University, Washington, DC

ALEXANDER G. PANOSSIAN, PhD, DSci
Head of Research and Development, Research and Development, Swedish Herbal Institute, Vallberga, Halland, Sweden

JEROME SARRIS, MHSc, PhD
NHMRC Clinical Research Fellow, Faculty of Medicine, Department of Psychiatry, The University of Melbourne, The Melbourne Clinic, Richmond; Centre for Human Psychopharmacology, Swinburne University of Technology, Hawthorn, Victoria, Australia

STUART N. SEIDMAN, MD
West End Medical Associates, New York, New York; Department of Psychiatry, Sheba Medical Center, Tel-Hashomer, Israel

LESLIE SHERLIN, PhD
Neurotopia, Inc, Marina Del Rey, California; Nova Tech EEG, Inc, Mesa; Arizona Brain Performance Center, Mesa; Adjunct Assistant Professor and Clinical Faculty, Southwest College of Naturopathic Medicine, Tempe; Faculty, University of Phoenix, Phoenix, Arizona

SUSAN B. SHOR, LCSW
Executive Director, Princeton Biofeedback Centre, Princeton, New Jersey

NILKAMAL SINGH, MSc
Senior Research Fellow, Department of Research on Yoga, Patanjali Research Foundation, Haridwar, Uttarakhand, India

SHIRLEY TELLES, MBBS, PhD (Neurophysiology)
Director of Research, Department of Research on Yoga, Patanjali Research Foundation, Haridwar, Uttarakhand, India

MARK WEISER, MD
Associate Professor and Chair, Department of Psychiatry, Sackler Faculty of Medicine, Tel Aviv University; Chief Psychiatrist, Department of Psychiatry, Sheba Medical Center, Tel-Hashomer, Israel

Contents

SECTION 1. NUTRIENTS

Folate (vitamin B$_9$) and cobalamin (vitamin B$_{12}$) are essential for the normal development and function of the central nervous system. The metabolism of these vitamins is intimately linked and supports the synthesis of S-adenosylmethionine (SAMe), the major methyl group donor in methylation reactions. This article reviews the metabolic and clinical importance of folate, vitamin B$_{12}$, and SAMe, as well as clinical trials in relation to depression and dementia.

Over the past 2 decades, omega-3 fatty acids (n-3FAs) have been increasingly used and studied in the United States and worldwide for various medical and psychiatric indications. Numerous published clinical trials have examined applications of different n-3FA preparations, primarily in mood disorders but also in psychotic disorders, attention-deficit disorder, obsessive-compulsive disorder, and personality disorders. Focusing on clinical issues, this article reviews the impact of n-3FAs on these conditions and covers the relevant research, side effects, dosage guidelines, and drug interactions; clinicians should thus be able to better advise patients who are already taking n-3FAs or are interested in trying them.

The choice of nutrients for review is based on clinical evidence of efficacy in neuropsychiatric disorders and biochemical effects that are neuroprotective or reparative. Vitamins, minerals, amino acids, and metabolites have been shown to augment antidepressants, improve symptoms in anxiety disorders, depression, neurodegenerative diseases, brain injury, ADHD, and schizophrenia, and to reduce medication side effects. Detection and correction of vitamin and mineral deficiencies can be essential for recovery. Generally low in adverse effects when taken in therapeutic doses, nutrients can be combined for greater benefits. Further studies are warranted to validate these promising treatments.

SECTION 2. HERBAL MEDICINES

> Herbal medicines supported by evidence of safety and efficacy in the treatment of anxiety, insomnia, fatigue, cognitive enhancement, mental focus, and sexual function are useful as monotherapies, multiherb combinations, and as adjuncts to prescription psychotropics. Relevant mechanisms of action and clinical guidelines for herbs in common use can assist clinicians who want to enhance treatment outcomes by integrating phytomedicinals into their treatment regimens. Research is needed to strengthen the evidence base and to expand the range of disorders that can be treated with herbal extracts. Studies of herbal genomic effects may lead to more targeted and effective treatments.

> This article focuses on the most extensively studied adaptogens: *Rhodiola rosea, Eleutherococcus senticosus,* and *Schisandra chinensis.* Clinical studies, evidence for stress-protective and simulative effects, and molecular mechanisms of action on metabolic and other processes regulated by the neuroendocrine system are discussed.

> St. John's wort (*Hypericum perforatum*) has been extensively studied and reviewed for its use in depression; however, there is less salient discussion on its clinical application for a range of other psychiatric disorders. This article outlines the current evidence of the efficacy of St John's wort in common psychiatric disorders, including major depression, bipolar depression, attention-deficit hyperactivity disorder, obsessive-compulsive disorder, social phobia, and somatization disorder. Mechanisms of action, including emerging pharmacogenetic data, safety, and clinical considerations are also detailed.

> *Ginkgo biloba* special extract (EGb761) is used in most randomized control trials. Indications include cognition and memory in Alzheimer disease, age-associated dementia, cerebral insufficiency, intermittent claudication, schizophrenia, and multi-infarct dementia. Dosages range from 80 to 720 mg/d for durations of 2 weeks to 2 years. Mechanisms of action include increasing cerebral blood flow, antioxidant and antiinflammatory effects, with antiplatelet effects attributed to flavone and terpene lactones. Possible interactions with monoamine oxidase inhibitors, alprazolam, haloperidol, warfarin, and nifedipine have been reported. Optimal dosage/duration, dose-response characteristics, drug interactions, bioavailability,

long-term effects, and optimal intervention timing should be the focus of future work.

on physiological parameters such as heart rate variability. The empirical literature indicates that technology-assisted breathing can be beneficial in mental health treatment, though it may not be appropriate for all individuals. Initial in-person training and evaluation can improve results.

Mindfulness meditation-based therapies are being increasingly used as interventions for psychiatric disorders. Mindfulness-based stress reduction (MBSR) and mindfulness-based cognitive therapy (MBCT) have been studied extensively. MBSR is beneficial for general psychological health and pain management. MBCT is recommended as an adjunctive treatment for unipolar depression. Both MBSR and MBCT have efficacy for anxiety symptoms. Informed clinicians can do much to support their patients who are receiving mindfulness training. This review provides information needed by clinicians to help patients maximize the benefits of mindfulness training and develop an enduring meditation practice.

This article describes the role of attention training and brainwave synchrony training in the resolution of stress- and pain-related symptoms. It describes the origin of Open Focus attention training as it was distilled from observations of space-generated brain wave activity. It provides a map of the various attentional styles and associated EEG activity.

Neurofeedback is a machine-mediated noninvasive treatment modality based on the analysis and "feeding back" of electroencephalogram brainwaves, which has shown efficacy with a variety of central nervous system–based problems. It has special application where patients have adverse reaction to psychopharmacologic treatments and psychotherapy, cognitive behavioral therapy, and dialectical behavior therapy have proved ineffective. Treatment modalities include active forms based on operant conditioning, involving a subject's response to stimuli. Neurofeedback is strong in clinical confirmations of efficacy (case studies) and has thus far limited controlled studies in the peer-reviewed journals.

Cranial electrotherapy stimulation is a prescriptive medical device that delivers a mild form of electrical stimulation to the brain for the treatment of anxiety, depression, and insomnia. It is supported by more than 40 years of research demonstrating its effectiveness in several mechanistic studies and greater than 100 clinical studies. Adverse effects are rare (<1%), mild, and self-limiting, consisting mainly of skin irritation under the electrodes and headaches. Often used as a stand-alone therapy, because results are usually seen from the first treatment, cranial electrotherapy stimulation may also be used as an adjunctive therapy.

SECTION 5. HORMONAL TREATMENTS

Age-associated hypothalamic-pituitary-gonadal (HPG) axis hypofunction, or partial androgen deficiency of the aging male, is thought to be responsible for various age-associated conditions such as reduced muscle and bone mass, mobility limitations, frailty, obesity, sleep apnea, cognitive impairment, sexual dysfunction, and depression. It has been difficult to establish consistent correlations between these symptoms and plasma testosterone levels in middle-aged men, but testosterone replacement does lead to improved muscle strength, bone density, and sexual function. This article focuses on the relationship between testosterone and mood in older men, and the treatment of age-related depression with exogenous testosterone.

SECTION 6. PREGNANCY

A discussion of pharmacologic and nonpharmacologic management of mental disorders in the pregnant woman is presented, with the focus on alternative health approaches and nutrition awareness. The article explores some considerations of modifiable risk factors thought to play a role in epigenetic manifestations of infant and child illness. Several case examples show the potential for integrative medicine in patients of reproductive age.

PSYCHIATRIC CLINICS OF NORTH AMERICA

FORTHCOMING ISSUES

Psychiatric Manifestations of Neurotoxins
Daniel E. Rusyniak, MD, and
Michael R. Dobbs, MD, *Editors*

Disaster Psychiatry
Craig Katz, MD, and Anand Pandya, MD,
Editors

Late Life Depression
W. Vaughn McCall, MD, *Editor*

RECENT ISSUES

December 2012
Forensic Psychiatry
Charles L. Scott, MD, *Editor*

September 2012
Schizophrenia
Peter F. Buckley, MD, *Editor*

June 2012
Addiction
Itai Danovitch, MD, and
John J. Mariani, MD, *Editors*

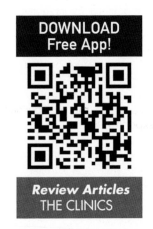

**DOWNLOAD
Free App!**

Review Articles
THE CLINICS

NOW AVAILABLE FOR YOUR iPhone and iPad

Preface

Along Roads Less Traveled: Complementary, Alternative, and Integrative Treatments

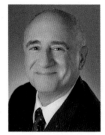
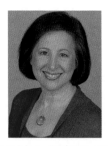
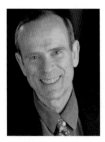

Philip R. Muskin, MD   Patricia L. Gerbarg, MD   Richard P. Brown, MD
Editors

Psychotropic medications have revolutionized the treatment of serious mental disorders, yet in a significant number of cases, they are partially effective or ineffective. Psychotropics are necessary for many patients but they can contribute to the burden of side effects, and the cost of psychotropics contributes to the cost of health care and disposal of these medications may cause environmental pollution. Phytomedicines, nutrients, and mind-body practices tend to be less costly and to have fewer side effects. Furthermore, much of the world's population has no access to prescription pharmaceuticals. Although psychotropics and psychotherapies will continue to be mainstays of psychiatric practice, specific combinations of herbs and nutrients can enhance the effectiveness of prescription drugs or reduce the necessary doses. Moreover, nutritional and phytomedicinal compounds can prevent or counteract various acute and long-term side effects of medications such as fatigue, Parkinsonian symptoms, akathisia, and elevated hepatic enzymes. Integrative psychiatrists are finding that mind-body practices can facilitate progress in psychotherapy. Identifying safe and effective nutrients, phytomedicines, and mind-body practices is therefore vital to better mental health care. Integrative treatments provide the clinician with additional therapeutic tools and empower the patient to participate actively in recovery.

We have invited authors to focus on treatments supported by an evidence base of significant benefits, associated with few and modest side effects. From the wide array of complementary, alternative, and integrative medicines (CAIM), we chose to include diverse points of view from experts who are well known, as well as from those whose work is not widely read by mainstream psychiatrists but who are highly regarded in their fields. The authors have been tasked with discussing the evidence base, neurophysiology, risks, benefits, and clinical applications for each treatment. Due to space limitations, commonly accepted and widely published treatments such as hypnosis

Psychiatr Clin N Am 36 (2013) xiii–xv
http://dx.doi.org/10.1016/j.psc.2013.01.009   **psych.theclinics.com**
0193-953X/13/$ – see front matter © 2013 Published by Elsevier Inc.

and acupuncture are not included. To accommodate as much content as possible, several authors have opted to allow the publisher to post most of their reference lists online, retaining only key references with their articles.

Modern research is rediscovering and improving on the benefits of nutrients, herbs, and mind-body practices. Every culture has used local medicinal plants whose active constituents can now being analyzed. The neurophysiologic changes that underlie psychiatric disorders involve multiple mechanisms, metabolites, anatomic structures, and neuro-endocrine networks. Nutrients and herbal extracts contain bioactive substances that can scavenge free radicals, protect cellular structures, enhance mitochondrial energy transport, increase production of neurotransmitters, upregulate or downregulate genes, and replenish vital metabolites. The rationale for integrating treatments is that targeting multiple etiologic factors often results in better outcomes than targeting only one, such as a particular neurotransmitter.

The scientific measurement of psycho-neuro-immuno-hormonal and genomic changes induced by mind-body practices opens a vast domain for treatments derived from spiritual, meditative, fitness, and brain stimulation techniques. Studies are finding that mind-body interventions can activate or mute neural networks involved in emotion regulation. Such interventions act to balance stress response systems, including the autonomic nervous system and the hypothalamic-pituitary-adrenal axis. Among thousands of mind-body practices, one can discern certain common healing elements, for example, breathing practices. Initially developed prior to 5000 BC in India as well as in Asia, Africa, Polynesia, and the Americas, these techniques reappeared in medieval monasteries and martial arts. Today such practices are used in yoga classes and in Special Forces training. It is not surprising that such time-tested treatments show significant clinical benefits in randomized controlled trials. Developing specific mind-body programs for various psychiatric conditions and treatment settings is an appealing future direction.

Political, economic, and environmental forces are driving large-scale natural and man-made disasters. Relying solely on expensive pharmaceuticals or one-on-one therapies will not address the global epidemic of depression and posttraumatic stress disorder. Affected populations need inexpensive, accessible, safe, sustainable treatments. The large-scale cultivation of medicinal herbs is increasing available supplies. Local teachers, care providers, clergy, and community leaders can be trained to provide and to train others in self-healing mind-body practices. Resiliency training could help at-risk communities prevent or recover from the psychological sequelae of traumatizing events. Mind-body programs could also enable members of the military to endure combat stress better and recover from service-related posttraumatic stress disorder.

Integrative psychiatry seeks to enrich mainstream mental health care with valuable treatments from global healing traditions as well as from modern laboratories in related fields, such as neurofeedback, breath pacing, and genomics. Interest, support, and research are growing, but much more is needed to strengthen the evidence base and to refine treatments for specific conditions. Educating ourselves, our peers, and our patients is essential for the safe and optimal use of CAIM approaches. This volume introduces treatments that the authors and editors deem to be worthy of consideration and future development. References provide avenues for further learning. As in any therapeutic endeavor, the journey starts with hearing what those who are experts have to say, followed by self-education and clinical experience. Along these less traveled roads, each of us has learned and used many of these methods successfully in treating patients who were unresponsive to standard approaches.

We wish to thank the authors for contributing their knowledge and experience to this volume. Elsevier also deserves appreciation for making available to their readership material not often included in mainstream publications.

Philip R. Muskin, MD
Columbia University Medical Center
Consultation-Liaison Psychiatry
NY-Presbyterian Hospital/Columbia Campus
622 W. 168th Street, Mailbox #427
New York, NY 10032, USA

Patricia L. Gerbarg, MD
New York Medical College
86 Sherry Lane
Valhalla, NY 12401, USA

Richard P. Brown, MD
Columbia University College of Physicians and Surgeons
30 East End Avenue
New York, NY 10028, USA

E-mail addresses:
prm1@columbia.edu (P.R. Muskin)
PGerbarg@aol.com (P.L. Gerbarg)
rpb1@columbia.edu (R.P. Brown)

Folate, Vitamin B$_{12}$, and S-Adenosylmethionine

Teodoro Bottiglieri, PhD

KEYWORDS

- Folate • Vitamin B$_{12}$ • S-adenosylmethionine • Methylation • Depression
- Dementia

KEY POINTS

- Folate is required in the synthesis of methionine and S-adenosylmethionine (SAMe). Folate deficiency is commonly associated with depression, but may also play an important role in cognitive function. Clinical trials with various forms of folate (folic acid, folinic acid, and 5-methyltetrahydrofolate) have provided evidence to support a therapeutic effect in these disorders.
- Vitamin B$_{12}$ is an essential cofactor required in 2 major pathways involving the synthesis of methionine that supports methylation and synthesis of succinyl-CoA, an intermediate of the citric acid cycle. Low vitamin B$_{12}$ levels are associated with depression and dementia. Supplementation with vitamin B$_{12}$ may protect against cognitive decline.
- SAMe, available as a dietary supplement, has been shown to have antidepressant properties. The mode of action of this compound may reside in its ability to upregulate monoamine metabolism.

OVERVIEW

There are similarities in the neuropsychiatric complications of folate (vitamin B$_9$) and cobalamin (vitamin B$_{12}$) deficiency, but the former is particularly associated with depression, especially in the elderly.[1,2] Moreover, extensive research in the last 30 years has demonstrated that folate and vitamin B$_{12}$ play essential roles in development and function of the central nervous system (CNS). This aspect is illustrated by the many cases of inherited disorders that impair uptake and metabolism of these vitamins, resulting in profound deleterious effects such as mental retardation, psychiatric disorders, seizures, and myelopathy.[3,4] A comparison of neuropsychiatric findings in patients with megaloblastic anemia caused by folate or vitamin B$_{12}$ deficiency (**Table 1**) shows that the most common finding associated with folate deficiency

Conflict of interest: Dr Bottiglieri reports having been the Chairman of the Advisory Board for Methylation Sciences Inc; holding stock options in Methylation Sciences Inc; is a Consultant for Gnosis S.P.A.; and having received grant/research funding from PamLab LLC, distributor of B vitamins as a medical food.
Institute of Metabolic Disease, Baylor Research Institute, Baylor University, 3812 Elm Street, Dallas, TX 75226, USA
E-mail address: teodorob@baylorhealth.edu

Psychiatr Clin N Am 36 (2013) 1–13
http://dx.doi.org/10.1016/j.psc.2012.12.001 psych.theclinics.com

Table 1
Neuropsychiatric findings in patients presenting with megaloblastic anemia

	Vitamin B_{12} Deficiency (N = 50)	Folic Acid Deficiency (N = 34)	P value
Neuropsychiatric Findings (%)			
Normal	32	35	NS
Cognitive change	26	27	NS
Affective disorder	20	56	<.001
Subacute combined degeneration	16	0	<.05
Peripheral neuropathy	40	18	<.1
Optic atrophy	2	0	NS
Cause of Anemia			
Pernicious anemia	32	—	
Dietary	8	8	
Gastrointestinal	7	—	
Celiac disease	—	16	
Malabsorption	—	8	
Unexplained	3	2	

Abbreviation: NS, not significant.
Data from Shorvon SD, Carney MW, Chanarin I, et al. The neuropsychiatry of megaloblastic anemia. Br Med J 1980;281(6247):1036–8.

was affective disorder (56%), whereas dementia and cognitive impairment were present in about one-quarter of both groups. The most common association with B_{12} deficiency was peripheral neuropathy (40%). Spinal cord demyelination (subacute combined degeneration) was noted in B_{12} deficiency but not in folate deficiency.[2] However, several subsequent case reports indicate that demyelination of the spinal cord can also be a consequence of severe folate deficiency.[5,6] Of interest is the finding that approximately one-third of subjects in both groups had no neuropsychiatric complications. Undoubtedly, the duration of the vitamin deficiency as well as dietary and genetic factors can play a role. More importantly, if left untreated CNS involvement will occur in all cases.

METABOLISM OF FOLATE, VITAMIN B_{12}, AND S-ADENOSYLMETHIONINE

The intimate relationship between the metabolism of folate and vitamin B_{12} can account for some of the similarities in clinical symptoms that occur when these vitamins are deficient or when their metabolism is disrupted. The metabolic interface between folate and vitamin B_{12} is the conversion of homocysteine (Hcy) to methionine (**Fig. 1**). This reaction, catalyzed by methionine synthase, requires a reduced form of folate, 5-methyltetrahydrofolate (5-MTHF), as well as vitamin B_{12}. Methionine, an essential amino acid, is the substrate for the synthesis of SAMe, an important metabolite that is the sole methyl group donor in more than 100 methylation reactions in the body.[7] Methylation, a vital biochemical process required for normal cell function, involves the transfer of a methyl group (CH_3) from the primary donor compound, SAMe, to an acceptor molecule. This process generates S-adenosylhomocysteine (SAH), which is metabolized to Hcy and completes the methylation cycle. Because Hcy is absent from any dietary source and is produced solely as a byproduct of the methylation cycle, the circulating blood level bound to protein, total

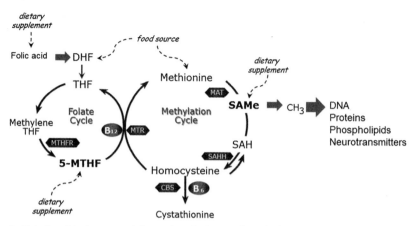

Fig. 1. Relationship between folate, vitamin B$_{12}$, and methylation. DHF, dihydrofolate; THF, tetrahydrofolate; 5-MTHF, 5-methyltetrahydrofolate; SAMe, *S*-adenosylmethionine; SAH, *S*-adenosylhomocysteine; MTHFR, methyltetrahydrofolate reductase; MTR, methioinine synthase; MAT, methionine adenosyltransferase; SAHH, *S*-adenosylhomocysteine hydrolase.

homocysteine (tHcy), is a sensitive indicator of both folate and vitamin B$_{12}$ deficiency, as well as the functional activity of the folate/methylation cycle.[8] Acceptor molecules in methylation-dependent reactions include DNA bases, proteins, phospholipids, neurotransmitters, free amino acids, and other compounds. DNA methylation controls the expression of genes and can turn the transcription of cellular proteins "on" or "off." Similarly, methylation of proteins results in posttranslational modifications that can influence enzyme activity. Methylation of phospholipids is necessary for cell-membrane integrity and optimal function of receptors that are localized in the lipid membrane bilayer. SAMe is the universal methyl donor in more than 100 methyltransferase reactions, which are catalyzed by specific methyltransferase enzymes and which modulate metabolic pathways.[7] It is not surprising, therefore, that aberrant methylation has been implicated as a pathogenic mechanism in CNS disorders, including depression and dementia,[9,10] and methyl-donor therapy has become a therapeutic target to prevent or delay disease progression and/or enhance clinical outcome.[9,11,12]

Vitamin B$_{12}$ is also an essential cofactor in the conversion of methylmalonyl coenzyme A (MMCoA) to succinyl coenzyme A, which is catalyzed by MMCoA mutase. This pathway is related to the catabolism of propionate, which is derived from the breakdown of odd-chain fatty acids. Vitamin B$_{12}$ deficiency leads to decreased activity of MMCoA mutase activity and elevated levels of methylmalonic acid (MMA) in blood and urine.[8] Measurement of MMA and homocysteine provides a functional measure of intracellular B$_{12}$ levels, and provides additional evidence with which to monitor the status of vitamin B$_{12}$.

FOLATE
Depression

Studies on the association of folate deficiency with depression initially conducted in epileptic patients showed that anticonvulsant treatment led to low levels of serum folate, resulting in a higher incidence of mental symptoms including depression and psychosis.[13] Between 1967 and 1990 all surveys of folate deficiency, including 16 studies in depression, mania, and schizophrenia, and 5 studies of psychogeriatric patients including dementia,[14] reported a high incidence of low levels of serum folate. A United States study of study of 213 depressed outpatients showed that subjects with low folate levels were less likely to respond to standard antidepressant treatment.[15] A general population study involving 2256 subjects without depression, 301 subjects with depression, and 121 subjects with dysthymia reported significant associations between levels of serum and red cell folate and depression.[16]

Despite numerous reports on the association between folate deficiency and depression, relatively few controlled clinical trials have investigated the effect of folate treatment alone (without other vitamins) on mood disorders. By contrast, numerous studies have investigated the effects of multivitamin complexes, typically a combination of folate, vitamin B_{12}, and vitamin B_6. In studies of folate alone, 6 clinical trials, 2 open and 4 double-blind controlled, have used different forms of folate; 2 trials used folic acid, 1 trial used folinic acid, and 3 trials used 5-MTHF. These studies are summarized in **Table 2**. All but 1 of the 6 trials used folate supplementation as an adjuvant to standard psychotropic medication.

One of the first double-blind randomized, placebo-controlled (DBRPC) trials evaluated the effect of a daily supplement of 200 µg folic acid or a matched placebo on affective morbidity in a group of 75 patients on lithium therapy.[17] This 1-year study showed that patients with the highest concentrations of plasma folate had a significant reduction in their affective morbidity. This finding led the investigators to suggest that a daily supplement of 300 to 400 µg/d folic acid could be useful in long-term lithium treatment. 5-MTHF, 15 mg/d improved depression in folate-deficient patients with major depression and schizophrenia being assessed at 3 and 6 months of therapy.[18]

In another large DBRPC trial involving 127 depressed patients, the effect of folic acid versus placebo given as an adjuvant to fluoxetine treatment was compared.[19] Significant reduction in Hamilton Depression Rating Scale (HAM-D) scores was observed in the folic acid + fluoxetine group, but only in female patients. Female patients had the highest plasma folate and significantly lower plasma tHcy values after treatment compared with baseline values.

In an open trial, the effect of leucovorin (folinic acid) at a dose of 15 to 30 mg/d was assessed in subjects with major depressive disorder who had an inadequate response to selective serotonin reuptake inhibitors (SSRIs). Adjunctive treatment with leucovorin significantly improved response (50% or greater reduction in Ham-D-17 scores) and remission in SSRI refractory depression.[20]

Recently the efficacy of 5-MTHF as an adjunctive therapy for SSRI-resistant depression was studied in 2 randomized, double-blind, parallel sequential trials.[21] The L-isomer form (L-methylfolate) was used in both trials for 30 days. Two primary outcome measures for both studies were the difference in response rates defined as a reduction of 50% or greater in HAM-D score, and a response as defined by a final HAM-D score or 7 or less. In trial 1, no significant difference between the L-methylfolate (7.5 mg) and placebo groups was observed. However in trial 2, L-methylfolate (15 mg) showed a significant increase in response rate and the difference in degree of improvement on the HAM-D score compared with placebo. In both trials, L-methylfolate was well tolerated, with no significant difference in side effects between treatment groups. The results of this study support the use of L-methylfolate as an adjunctive treatment for SSRI-resistant depression, although this effect remains to be confirmed for other classes of antidepressants.

Dementia

Deficiencies of folate and vitamin B_{12} are common in the elderly population, and several studies have shown associations between the status of these vitamins and

Table 2
Clinical trials of folate supplementation in depression

Authors,[Ref.] Year	Design	Folate Supplement	Characteristics	Outcome
Coppen et al,[17] 1986	Double-blind randomized placebo-controlled 12 mo	Folic acid (200 μg) or placebo in combination with lithium	75 patients on lithium therapy	Patients with highest plasma folate had a greater reduction in affective morbidity
Godfrey et al,[18] 1990	Double-blind randomized placebo-controlled 6 mo	MTHF (15 mg) or placebo. Other psychotropic medication allowed	24 depressed and 17 schizophrenic DSM-III with low red cell folate <200 ng/mL	Significant decrease in mean outcome scores in MTHF group at 3 and 6 mo
Guaraldi et al,[57] 1993	Open trial 6 wk	MTHF (50 mg). No other psychotropic medication	20 elderly depressed subjects. DSM-III-R, HAM-D-21 ≥18	16 completed at least 4 wk 81% response rate (decreased HAM-D >50%)
Passeri et al,[58] 1993	Double-blind controlled 8 wk	MTHF (50 mg) or trazodone (100 mg). Other psychotropic medication allowed	96 patients with dementia, MMSE 12-23, and depression HAM-D >18	Significant decrease in HAM-D scores at 4 and 8 wk in MTHF and trazodone groups
Coppen and Bailey,[19] 2000	Double-blind randomized placebo-controlled 10 wk	Folic acid (500 μg) or placebo in combination with fluoxetine (20 mg)	127 depressed subjects DSM-III-R, HAM-D-17 ≥20	Significantly greater improvement in folic acid + fluoxetine group in females only. Effect linked to higher plasma folate and lower tHcy levels
Alpert et al,[20] 2002	Open trial 8 wk	Folinic acid in combination with an SSRI	22 depressed adults DSM-IV, HAM-D-17 ≥12. Partial or no response to an SSRI	16 completed 31% response rate (decreased HAM-D >50%), 19% remission
Papakostas et al,[21] 2012	Double-blind randomized placebo-controlled, of 2 parallel sequential trials 30 d	L-MTHF (trial 1 = 7.5 mg; trial 2 = 15 mg) or placebo as adjunctive therapy to SSRI	Treatment-resistant depressed patients Trial 1, N = 148 Trial 2, N = 75	In trial 1 L-MTHF (7.5 mg) had no significant difference. In trial 2 L-MTHF (15 mg) showed significantly greater response rate and degree of change in HAM-D score

Abbreviations: DSM, Diagnostic and Statistical Manual of Mental Disorders; HAM-D, Hamilton Depression Rating Scale; MTHF, 5-methyltetrahydrofolate; SSRI, selective serotonin reuptake inhibitor; tHcy, total homocysteine.

elevated levels of plasma tHcy regarding cognitive function.[22,23] Trials have been conducted to determine whether B-vitamin supplementation can improve cognitive function, in most cases using a combination of folic acid, vitamin B_{12}, and vitamin B_6. This treatment is intended to lower plasma concentrations of tHcy (a sulfur amino acid that is potentially toxic to vascular and neural cells), and to increase folate metabolism and synthesis of SAMe. **Table 3** summarizes the main large double-blind randomized controlled trials (DBRCTs) with a duration of 18 months or greater that have investigated the effect of folate and B vitamins on cognitive function in community-dwelling older subjects and in elderly subjects with mild cognitive impairment or Alzheimer dementia.

One trial found that 800 µg folic acid only, given daily for 3 years to community-dwelling men and women (age 50–70 years), improved measures of information processing and sensorimotor speed compared with placebo.[24]

In another study healthy subjects with no cognitive impairment, but with elevated plasma tHcy (>13 µM) were treated for 2 years with folic acid, vitamin B_{12}, and vitamin B_6. Despite a reduction in plasma tHcy, no effect on cognitive function was observed in the active treatment group.[25]

A more recent study of community-dwelling subjects with psychological stress showed significant improvement in cognitive function after 2 years of treatment with folic acid, vitamin B_{12}, and vitamin B_6.[26] Because a combination of folate, vitamin B_{12}, and vitamin B_6 was used, the extent of a synergistic effect is unclear.

Two DBRPC trials of folate and B vitamins in subjects with Alzheimer dementia failed to show any significant effect on cognitive function (see **Table 3**). However, in one study a planned subgroup Alzheimer Disease Assessment Scale—Cognitive Subscale (ADAS-cog) change analysis of subjects above and below the median Mini Mental State Examination (MMSE) score at baseline favored placebo in the lower MMSE group, but significantly favored active treatment in the higher MMSE group after 15 months.[27]

In summary, folate and B-vitamin treatment may slow the rate of cognitive decline (ADAS-cog change) in subjects less severely affected at baseline. In keeping with this observation, supplementation trials with folic acid, vitamin B_{12}, and B_6 in subjects with mild cognitive impairment (MCI) showed significant benefit in global cognition, episodic memory and semantic memory.[28] This benefit was significant in subjects with baseline plasma tHcy concentrations above the median (>11.3 µM). In a 24-month study folic acid and B vitamins significantly slowed the rate of brain atrophy in subjects with MCI, an effect that was also related to baseline plasma tHcy concentrations.[29]

Mechanism of Action

Folic acid is a synthetic form of folate that is absorbed and converted to reduced forms of folate such as formyl-tetrahydrofolate (folinic acid) or 5-MTHF. Active uptake of folate across the blood-brain-barrier occurs at specific folate-receptor α (FR-α) sites, localized in the choroid plexus. FR-α has a high affinity for 5-MTHF and a lower affinity for other reduced folates.[30] Once 5-MTHF enters the cerebrospinal fluid (CSF) compartment it is transported into neuronal cells, and participates in methylation of Hcy and synthesis of methionine and SAMe. By providing a source of methyl groups folate can support DNA, protein, phospholipid, and other methylation-dependent pathways implicated in depression and dementia.[10,31] In addition, 5-MTHF is involved in the biosynthesis of tetrahydrobiopterin, a rate-limiting cofactor for the synthesis of monoamine neurotransmitters[32] implicated in the pathophysiology of depression.

Table 3
Double-blind, randomized controlled trials of folate and B-vitamin supplementation on cognitive function

Authors,[Ref.] Year	Design	Folate Supplement	Characteristics	Outcome
Trials in Community-Dwelling Subjects				
McMahon et al,[25] 2006	Double-blind randomized placebo-controlled	Folic acid (1 mg) + vitamin B$_6$ (10 mg) + vitamin B$_{12}$ (0.5 mg) or placebo	276 healthy subjects, >65 y with elevated plasma tHcy (>13 μM)	No significant effect on cognitive measures in the folic acid group
Durga et al,[24] 2007	Double-blind randomized placebo-controlled 36 mo	Folic acid (800 mg) or placebo	818 community-dwelling men and women aged 50–70 y	Significant change in memory, speed of information processing, sensorimotor speed
Walker et al,[26] 2012	Double-blind randomized placebo-controlled 24 mo	Folic acid (400 mg) + vitamin B$_{12}$ (100 mg) or placebo	900 community-dwelling adults aged 60–74 y with elevated psychological distress	Improvement in cognitive function at 24 mo
Trials in Mild Cognitive Impairment or Alzheimer Dementia Subjects				
Aisen et al,[27] 2008	Double-blind randomized placebo-controlled 18 mo	Folic acid (5 mg) + vitamin B$_6$ (25 mg) + vitamin B$_{12}$ (1 mg) or placebo	340 subjects with Alzheimer disease. 202 active treatment and 138 placebo	High-dose B vitamins did not slow cognitive decline. Analysis of subjects above and below median on baseline MMSE showed significant effect in the higher MMSE group
Kwok et al,[60] 2011	Double-blind randomized placebo-controlled 24 mo	Folic acid (5 mg) + vitamin B$_{12}$ (1 mg) or placebo	140 subjects with mild to moderate Alzheimer disease	No significant effect on global cognitive decline
Smith et al,[29] 2010	Double-blind randomized placebo-controlled 24 mo	Folic acid (0.8 mg) + vitamin B$_6$ (20 mg) + vitamin B$_{12}$ (0.5 mg) or placebo	168 subjects with MCI over 70 y. 85 B vitamins, 83 placebo	Rate of brain atrophy in MCI patients slowed significantly by B vitamins. Effect related to baseline plasma tHcy
de Jager et al,[28] 2012	Double-blind randomized placebo-controlled 24 mo	Folic acid (0.8 mg) + vitamin B$_6$ (20 mg) + vitamin B$_{12}$ (0.5 mg) or placebo	266 subjects with MCI over 70 y. 133 B vitamins, 133 placebo	Significant benefit in subjects with baseline plasma tHcy above median in global cognition, episodic memory, semantic memory

Abbreviations: Hcy, homocysteine; MCI, mild cognitive impairment; MMSE, Mini Mental State Examination.

VITAMIN B$_{12}$
Depression

Vitamin B$_{12}$ deficiency has been reported in numerous studies to be associated with psychiatric disorders including depression, bipolar disorder, panic disorder psychosis, and phobias.[1,2] Symptoms that may precede a psychiatric diagnosis in such cases include agitation, irritability, negativism, confusion, disorientation, amnesia, impaired concentration and attention, and insomnia. Several cross-sectional studies in community-dwelling elderly subjects indicate that vitamin B$_{12}$ deficiency is independently associated with depression.

In one study in the Netherlands, 278 individuals older than 55 years with depressive symptoms had lower levels of plasma vitamin B$_{12}$.[33]

In Chinese elderly subjects (n = 669) a low level of vitamin B$_{12}$ (<180 pmol/L) was significantly associated with depressive symptoms (odds ratio 2.68), independent of folate or tHcy levels.[34]

These findings are consistent with an earlier study of 700 community-dwelling older women that found a 2-fold risk of severe depression in subjects with elevated MMA levels (a marker of B$_{12}$ deficiency).[35] However, one randomized placebo-controlled trial in elderly men did not find that vitamin B$_{12}$ supplementation for 2 years had any significant effect in reducing severity or incidence of depressive symptoms.[36] Most studies suggest that supplementation with vitamin B$_{12}$ may play a role in the treatment of depression. A prospective study of 115 outpatients with major depressive disorder showed that higher vitamin B$_{12}$ levels correlate with a better response to treatment.[37] Also, several case reports describe a lack of antidepressant response in individuals with vitamin B$_{12}$ deficiency who showed considerable clinical improvement following supplementation with vitamin B$_{12}$.[38,39]

There is no current recommended guideline for the prophylactic use of vitamin B$_{12}$ in the treatment of depression. Side effects of vitamin B$_{12}$ are rare. One report found that a combination of folate, B$_6$, and B$_{12}$ supplementation increased the risk of restenosis by 8% in men only with cardiac stents and a baseline Hcy of less than 15 μmol/L.[40] Considering the low level of adverse effects, clinicians may choose to prescribe vitamin B$_{12}$ in depressed patients or in those with low serum levels of vitamin B$_{12}$ or elevated MMA.

Dementia

There is a strong association between vitamin B$_{12}$ deficiency, cognitive impairment, and dementia. The best example can be found in patients with pernicious anemia who develop a dementia syndrome that responds well to vitamin B$_{12}$ treatment, when given before irreversible damage occurs.[1,41] The relationship between low levels of serum vitamin B$_{12}$ and cognitive function in healthy elderly subjects has been extensively studied, and the symptoms described can often overlap with those observed in dementia of the Alzheimer type. Furthermore, low serum vitamin B$_{12}$ has been associated with greater cognitive impairment in patients with Alzheimer disease. This association is stronger when elevated plasma tHcy is present, which has been shown to be a risk factor for dementia.[29,41]

Mechanism of Action

Vitamin B$_{12}$ is an essential cofactor for 2 enzymes, namely methionine synthase and MMCoA mutase. High doses can help maintain low blood levels of Hcy and MMA. Vitamin B$_{12}$–dependent metabolism of Hcy to methionine enhances SAMe synthesis and methylation in the same manner as folate. In addition, maintaining low levels of

MMA helps prevent abnormal fatty acid synthesis that can affect the neuronal membrane.[42]

S-ADENOSYLMETHIONINE
Depression

Clinical studies starting in the 1970s indicated that SAMe had antidepressant effects. Over the next 2 decades, the efficacy of SAMe in treating depressive disorders was confirmed in more than 40 clinical trials. In a meta-analysis, Bressa[43] reviewed 25 controlled trials including a total of 791 patients. This analysis concluded that SAMe had a significantly greater response rate than placebo and was comparable with tricyclic antidepressants. Brown and colleagues[44] summarized the literature on the use of SAMe in depressive disorders and reported that SAMe had been studied in 16 open, uncontrolled trials (660 patients); 13 DBRCTs (537 patients); and 19 controlled trials comparing SAMe with other antidepressants (1134 patients). Significant antidepressant effects were observed in all 16 open trials. In 18 controlled trials, SAMe was as effective as chlorimipramine, imipramine, and nomifensine. In these studies SAMe had far fewer side effects than standard medications. Carpenter[45] summarized clinical trials of intravenous or intramuscular formulations of SAMe in the treatment of mild to moderate depression (**Table 4**), and moderate to severe depression (**Table 5**).

More recent studies have focused on an oral formulation of SAMe that was introduced as a dietary supplement in the United States in 1998, and marketed for mood and emotional well-being. A DBRCT of SAMe tablets, similar to the over-the-counter dietary supplement, was administered to 73 serotonin reuptake inhibitor (SRI) nonresponders with major depressive disorders.[46] The adjunctive oral dose of SAMe (800 mg twice daily) was shown to augment the response rates for depression at the end of the 6-week trial. In this study the dose of SAMe was both effective and well tolerated. The United States Agency for Healthcare Research and Quality issued an evidence report based on a systematic review of SAMe research. The report found no statistically significant difference in outcomes between patients treated with SAMe and those on prescription antidepressants, but SAMe caused fewer side effects.[12] SAMe was also as effective as nonsteroidal anti-inflammatory medications in treating osteoarthritic pain, but had fewer gastrointestinal side effects. Studies also showed SAMe to be effective for relief of pruritus and for reducing elevated serum bilirubin levels associated with cholestasis of pregnancy. SAMe thus provides dual benefits in depressed patients with osteoarthritis or liver problems.

In an 8-week DBRPC study of 18 schizophrenic patients, oral SAMe (800 mg/d) significantly improved depression and ameliorated aggressive symptoms.[4] Oral SAMe treatment for 8 weeks was also significantly reduced depressive symptoms in 20 patients seropositive for human immunodeficiency virus who were diagnosed with major depressive disorder.[48]

Most trials of oral SAMe have been performed in patients with major depressive disorder. One limitation is that relatively small numbers of subjects (fewer than 50 patients in each therapeutic arm) were recruited into DBRCTs (see **Tables 4** and **5**). The dose of oral SAMe in these studies varies from 800 to 1600 mg daily. In one study involving treatment-resistant depression in patients with Parkinson disease, the dose of SAMe was titrated up from 800 mg to a maximum of 3600 mg per day to obtain response in some patients, without any serious adverse effects.[49] Treatment of Parkinson disease with Levodopa depletes SAMe supplies in the brain, causing depression, a condition that is reversed by high-dose SAMe supplementation. However, the literature lacks dose-escalation studies for the treatment of depression

Table 4
Randomized controlled studies of SAMe in the treatment of mild to moderate depression

Authors,[Ref.] Year	Treatment Arms	Mean Baseline HAM-D (±SD)	Study Duration	Primary Outcome	Primary Efficacy Results/ P Value (SAMe vs Placebo) Positive	Negative	Effect Size
Agnoli et al,[61] 1976	a. SAMe 15 mg IM TID; n = 20 b. Placebo; n = 10	21.6 (1.26) 19.1 (2.42)	15 d	HAM-D total change	<.05		1.6
Fava et al,[62] 1992	a. SAMe 1600 mg/d PO; n = 17 b. Placebo; n = 21	27.2a (4.8) 24.6a (4.3)	6 wk	HAM-D total change		NS	0.16
Thomas et al,[63] 1987	a. SAMe 200 mg/d IV; n = 9 b. Placebo; n = 11	26.6b (4.2) 25.2b (4.6)	2 wk	HAM-D total change		NS	0.12
Salmaggi et al,[64] 1993	a. SAMe 1600 mg/d PO; n = 40 b. Placebo; n = 40	24.4b (3.0) 23.5b (3.0)	30 d	HAM-D total change	<.01		0.33
De Leo,[65] 1987	a. SAMe 200 mg IM QD; n = 20 b. Placebo; n = 20	NAV	4 wk	Zung Self-Rating Depression Scale	<.05		0.61
Anacarani et al,[66] 1993	a. SAMe 400 mg/QOD IV; n = 41 b. Placebo; n = 10	25.73b (8.58) 20.66b (8.60)	3 wk	IPAT-DS change	P value for comparison between groups not provided		NAV
Cerutti et al,[67] 1993	a. SAMe 1600 mg/d PO; n = 30 b. Placebo; n = 30	NAV	30 d	Kellner Symptom Questionnaire	P value for comparison between groups not provided		NAV
Janicak et al,[68] 1989	a. SAMe 400 mg/d IV; n = 7 b. Imipramine 150 mg/d IV; n = 3 c. Placebo; n = 5	33.6a (9.0) 33.3a (6.9) 32.9a (5.9)	15 d	HAM-D total change	<.02		1.46
Carrieri et al,[69] 1990	2 period crossover design: a. SAMe 1000 mg/d→placebo; n = 11 b. Placebo→SAMe 1000 mg/d; n = 10	~26b (NAV) ~24b (NAV)	15 d (per crossover arm)	HAM-D total change	<.05		NAV

Based on the 17 item HAM-D unless otherwise specified.
Abbreviations: IM, intramuscular; IPAT-DS, Personality and Ability Testing—Depression Scale; IV, intravenous; NAV, no data available; PO, by mouth; QD, every day; QOD, every other day; TID, 3 times daily.
a Based on the 24-item HAM-D.
b Based on the 21-item HAM-D.
Data from Carpenter DJ. St. John's wort and S-adenosyl methionine as "natural" alternatives to conventional antidepressants in the era of the suicidality boxed warning: what is the evidence for clinically relevant benefit? Altern Med Rev 2011;16(1):17–39.

with SAMe. Current evidence suggests that in clinical trials the lowest dose of SAMe shown to be effective is 800 mg/d for mild to moderate depression and 1600 mg/d for severe major depressive disorder.

Dementia

The effect of SAMe on age-related cognitive decline or dementia has not been extensively studied. Despite the lack of large well-controlled clinical trials, there is significant evidence to support a role of SAMe and methylation in dementia. Concentrations of SAMe in CSF have been reported to be significantly reduced in Alzheimer dementia[50,51] and administration of oral SAMe for 3 to 5 months (400 mg 3 times daily), can increase plasma and CSF concentrations and improve measures of cognitive function as well as mood and speed of mental processing.[52] In a more recent DBRPC study on the use of adjunctive SAMe in 47 patients with major depressive disorder, a secondary analysis demonstrated that oral SAMe (1600 mg daily) improved memory-related cognitive symptoms such as the ability to recall information and word finding.[53]

Mechanism of Action

In relation to depression, preclinical studies in animal models have demonstrated that SAMe administration can increase the concentration of the monoamine neurotransmitters, serotonin and norepinephrine, in brain tissue. In humans, administration of oral SAMe (800 mg daily) for 2 weeks significantly increased concentrations of 5-hydroxyindoleacetic acid in CSF, a marker for increased serotonin in the brain.[50] The stimulatory effect of SAMe on central monoaminergic neurotransmitters is a likely viable mechanism underlying its antidepressant effect. There is a modest body of literature linking hypomethylation as a major biological mechanism involved in the etiology of dementia. This evidence includes reports of decreased SAMe concentrations in CSF in patients with Alzheimer disease,[50,51] increased concentrations of SAH in brain tissue, an inhibitor of methylation reactions,[54] hypomethylation of proteins that regulate levels of brain tissue phosphorylated-Tau,[31,55] and hypomethylation of genes that affect the expression of β-amyloid protein.[10,56] The effect of SAMe on site-specific methylation of DNA-promoter regions that regulate gene function, and carboxymethylation of proteins that can regulate β-amyloid and phosphorylation of Tau proteins is important, because these are well-established neuropathological hallmarks of Alzheimer disease.

S-Adenosylmethionine in Clinical Practice: Product Quality, Benefits, Risks, Hepatoprotection, Medication Interactions

Because SAMe is rapidly oxidized when exposed to air, the quality of the tablets is important in preserving potency.[44] "Bargain brands" marketed on the Internet and through stores often contain inactive isomers. Tablets must be preserved in individual blister packs that should not be refrigerated. Pharmaceutical grade SAMe is available from Europe.[44] SAMe is better absorbed when taken at least 20 minutes before breakfast and 20 minutes before lunch. As an activating antidepressant, it can disturb sleep if taken after 4:00 PM.

Unlike many prescription antidepressants, SAMe does not cause weight gain, sexual dysfunction, sedation, or cognitive interference. The most common side effects are gastrointestinal: nausea, loose bowels, diarrhea, abdominal discomfort and, rarely, vomiting. Patients who are sensitive to activation may feel jittery, overstimulated, anxious, or agitated. It is sometimes necessary to use a calming agent until this overactivation subsides. Less common side effects are headache or palpitations in patients with preexisting arrhythmias. SAMe is contraindicated in patients with

Table 5
Randomized, controlled studies of SAMe in the treatment of moderate to severe depression

Authors,[Ref.] Year	Treatment Arms	Mean Baseline HAM-D (±SD)	Study Duration	Primary Outcome	Primary Efficacy Results/*P* Value (SAMe vs Placebo) Positive	Negative	Effect Size
Kagan et al,[70] 1990	a. SAMe 1600 mg/d PO; n = 9 b. Placebo; n = 6	26.6[a] (5.5) 31.0[a] (8.5)	3 wk	HAM-D total change	<.05		0.79
Caruso et al,[71] 1987	a. SAMe 200 mg IM QD; n = 30 b. Placebo; n = 30	45.1[b] (6.7) 42.4[b] (5.1)	3 wk	HAM-D total change	<.01		1.4
Delle Chiale and Boissard,[72] 1997	a. SAMe 800 mg IV; n = 40 b. Placebo; n = 35	29.9 (4.0) 30.0 (3.2)	3 wk	HAM-D total change	<.05		0.43
Muscettola et al,[73] 1982	a. SAMe 150 mg IM QD; n = 10 b. Placebo; n = 10	23.2[c] (NAV) 22.2[c] (NAV)	15 d	HAM-D total change	<.5		NAV
Carney et al,[74] 1986	a. SAMe 200 mg IV; n = 16 b. Placebo; n = 16	26.5[a] (5.3) 25.5[a] (5.7)	2 wk	HAM-D total change		NS	0.36

Based on the 17-item HAM-D unless otherwise specified.
[a] Based on the 21-item HAM-D.
[b] Based on the 28-item HAM-D.
[c] Based on the 14-item HAM-D.
Data from Carpenter DJ. St. John's wort and *S*-adenosyl methionine as "natural" alternatives to conventional antidepressants in the era of the suicidality boxed warning: what is the evidence for clinically relevant benefit? Altern Med Rev 2011;16(1):17–39.

bipolar disorder because it can induce mania. SAMe has been found to reduce adverse hepatic effects from alcohol abuse, medications (including antidepressants and antiepileptics),[57] infection, and other causes. When SSRIs induce elevated liver-function tests, switching to SAMe will accelerate normalization of liver enzymes while treating the depression. A few case reports found SAMe to be safe and effective in children with severe chronic depressions, but to date no controlled trials have been completed in children.

The usual starting dose is 400 mg/d with increases every 5 to 7 days to a maximum of 800 mg twice daily. Improvements usually begin within 10 days, but may take several weeks. Elderly, frail, or sensitive patients may need to absorb the increase more gradually in 200-mg increments. If the patient does not respond after 4 weeks, doses may be increased by 400 mg/d every 1 to 2 weeks. On rare occasion, doses above 2000 mg are needed for depression.

ACKNOWLEDGMENTS

The author wishes to thank Dr Patricia Gerberg for her critical review and invaluable contributions to this article.

APPENDIX: REFERENCES

The complete reference list is online at http://www.psych.theclinics.com/dx.doi.org/10.1016/j.psc.2012.12.001.

KEY REFERENCES

2. Shorvon SD, Carney MW, Chanarin I, et al. The neuropsychiatry of megaloblastic anaemia. Br Med J 1980;281(6247):1036–8.
9. Bottiglieri T. S-Adenosyl-L-methionine (SAMe): from the bench to the bedside molecular basis of a pleiotrophic molecule. Am J Clin Nutr 2002;76(5):1151S–7S.
12. Hardy ML, Coulter I, Morton SC, et al. S-adenosyl-L-methionine for treatment of depression, osteoarthritis, and liver disease. Evid Rep Technol Assess (Summ.) 2003;64:1–3.
14. Crellin R, Bottiglieri T, Reynolds EH. Folates and psychiatric disorders. Clinical potential. Drugs 1993;45(5):623–36.
24. Durga J, van Boxtel MP, Schouten EG, et al. Effect of 3-year folic acid supplementation on cognitive function in older adults in the FACIT trial: a randomised, double blind, controlled trial. Lancet 2007;369(9557):208–16.
27. Aisen PS, Schneider LS, Sano M, et al. Alzheimer Disease Cooperative Study. High-dose B vitamin supplementation and cognitive decline in Alzheimer disease: a randomized controlled trial. JAMA 2008;300(15):1774–83.
29. Smith AD, Smith SM, de Jager CA, et al. Homocysteine-lowering by B vitamins slows the rate of accelerated brain atrophy in mild cognitive impairment: a randomized controlled trial. PLoS One 2010;5(9):e12244.
32. Stahl SM. L-methylfolate: a vitamin for your monoamines. J Clin Psychiatry 2008;69(9):1352–3.
44. Brown R, Gerberg P, Bottiglieri T. S-Adenosylmethionine in the clinical practice of psychiatry, neurology and internal medicine. Clin Pract Intern Med 2000;1:230–41.
45. Carpenter DJ. St. John's wort and S-adenosyl methionine as "natural" alternatives to conventional antidepressants in the era of the suicidality boxed warning: what is the evidence for clinically relevant benefit? Altern Med Rev 2011;16(1):17–39.

Omega-3 Fatty Acids in Psychiatry

David Mischoulon, MD, PhD[a,b,*], Marlene P. Freeman, MD[b,c]

KEYWORDS

- Omega-3 • n-3 • Depression • Bipolar disorder
- Complementary and alternative medicine • Ethyl-eicosapentaenoate
- Docosahexaenoic acid

KEY POINTS

- Omega-3 fatty acids (n-3FAs) are widely used for the treatment of various psychiatric conditions, particularly major depressive disorder and bipolar disorder.
- Eicosapentaenoic acid (EPA) and docosahexaenoic acid (DHA), derived from fish oil, are the n-3FAs that seem to be most important in terms of psychiatric disorders and in other fields of medicine.
- Recommended doses for depressive disorders are typically 1000–2000 mg/day of an EPA/DHA combination, preferably at an EPA:DHA ratio of 3:2 or greater.
- Dosing recommendations for other psychiatric disorders are less clear, due to limited and conflicting data.
- Adverse effects from n-3FAs may include minor gastrointestinal upset, cycling in bipolar patients, and a theoretical risk of bleeding when combined with anticoagulant drugs such as warfarin or aspirin.

OVERVIEW

Dietary intake of omega-3 fatty acids (n-3FAs) in Western society has decreased dramatically over the past century while the intake of processed foods rich in vegetable oils containing omega-6 (n-6) has increased. This dietary shift has resulted in a higher physiologic ratio of n-6:n-3 fatty acids in Western countries compared with countries with higher fish and n-3 consumption.[1–5] The modern Western diet, coupled with the increasingly stressful twenty-first century life, have been postulated to create a proinflammatory state in humans that is thought to contribute to cardiovascular and psychiatric illness.[6] Administration of n-3FA supplements may potentially reverse this

[a] Depression Clinical and Research Program, Massachusetts General Hospital, Harvard Medical School, 1 Bowdoin Square, 6th Floor, Boston, MA 02114, USA; [b] Department of Psychiatry, Massachusetts General Hospital, Harvard Medical School, Boston, MA, USA; [c] Perinatal and Reproductive Psychiatry Program, Harvard Medical School, Simches 2, 185 Cambridge Street, Boston, MA 02114, USA
* Corresponding author. Massachusetts General Hospital, 1 Bowdoin Square, 6th Floor, Boston, MA 02114.
E-mail address: dmischoulon@partners.org

Psychiatr Clin N Am 36 (2013) 15–23
http://dx.doi.org/10.1016/j.psc.2012.12.002
0193-953X/13/$ – see front matter © 2013 Elsevier Inc. All rights reserved.

proinflammatory state by correcting the n-6FA:n-3FA ratio, thus providing beneficial cardiovascular and psychiatric effects.

Over the past 2 decades, research on n-3FAs in psychiatry has included many treatment studies with encouraging evidence of clinical efficacy for n-3 in mood disorders (unipolar depression and bipolar disorder), and more preliminary data on conditions such as psychotic disorders and personality disorders. The 2 n-3 fatty acids most relevant to psychiatry are eicosapentaenoic acid (EPA; 20:5) and docosahexaenoic acid (DHA; 22:6), both of which are found primarily in fish oil and other marine sources (**Fig. 1**). Other important fatty acids include the shorter-chain n-3FAs such as α-linolenic acid (ALA; 18:3), obtained from flaxseed and other plants, although the evidence for ALA as a psychotropic is scant.[7] Linoleic acid (LA; 18:2) and the n-6 arachidonic acid (AA; 20:4) are also of interest; for example, the proinflammatory AA is reported to be displaced by EPA and DHA supplementation, suggesting a competitive dynamic between them that may account for some of the beneficial effects of n-3FAs.[8] As of this writing, most clinical investigations of psychotropic efficacy have examined EPA and DHA separately and in combination with each other, with a paucity of research on other essential fatty acids.

PROPOSED MECHANISMS OF PSYCHOTROPIC ACTION

n-3FAs may exert antidepressant effects through a variety of possible mechanisms of action. Proposed mechanisms of n-3FAs for the amelioration of mood disorders include an effect on membrane-bound receptors and enzymes involved in the regulation of neurotransmitter signaling, including increased serotonergic neurotransmission[9,10] and alterations in dopaminergic function,[11,12] as well as regulation of calcium-ion influx through calcium channels.[6] This process may contribute to stabilization and fluidity of neuronal membranes. Interaction with nuclear receptors has also been proposed.[6] Hamazaki and colleagues[13] found that administration of a combination of EPA and DHA to healthy subjects resulted in a lowering of plasma norepinephrine levels in comparison with placebo, suggesting that n-3FAs could exert their effect by interaction with catecholamines.

Omega-3 administration may counter the impact of n-6FA–derived eicosanoids and inhibit secretion of inflammatory cytokines, resulting in decreased corticosteroid release from the adrenal gland and dampening of the mood-altering effects associated with cortisol.[6,14] For example, EPA inhibits the synthesis of prostaglandin E_2, thus reducing the synthesis of P-glycoprotein, the latter of which may be involved in

---

Docosahexaenoic acid (DHA)

$CH_3\text{-}CH_2\text{-}CH=CH\text{-}CH_2\text{-}CH=CH\text{-}CH_2\text{-}CH=CH\text{-}CH_2\text{-}CH=CH\text{-}CH_2\text{-}CH=CH\text{-}CH_2\text{-}CH=CH\text{-}CH_2\text{-}CH_2\text{-}COOH$

Docosahexaenoic acid (22:6, n-3) has a 22-carbon chain and six double bonds. The leftmost carbon is termed the "omega" carbon, and the first double bond occurs on the third carbon from the left, hence the term "omega-3."

Eicosapentaenoic acid (EPA)

$CH_3\text{-}CH_2\text{-}CH=CH\text{-}CH_2\text{-}CH=CH\text{-}CH_2\text{-}CH=CH\text{-}CH_2\text{-}CH=CH\text{-}CH_2\text{-}CH=CH\text{-}CH_2\text{-}CH2\text{-}CH_2\text{-}COOH$

Eicosapentaenoic acid (20:5, n-3) has a 20-carbon chain and five double bonds. The first double bond occurs on the third carbon from the left.

Fig. 1. Docosahexaenoic acid (DHA) and eicosapentaenoic acid (EPA). (*From* Mischoulon D. Update and critique of natural remedies as antidepressant treatments. Obstet Gynecol Clin North Am 2009;36:789–807. Box 2; with permission.)

antidepressant resistance.[14] In this regard EPA resembles amitriptyline, which also inhibits P-glycoprotein and is generally considered useful for depression, particularly for treatment-resistant depression.

CLINICAL EFFICACY IN PSYCHIATRIC DISORDERS

Within psychiatry, n-3FAs have been studied most often in mood disorders and, to a lesser degree, in schizophrenia. More than 30 controlled trials and a few open studies in the United States with EPA and/or DHA suggest that supplementation with n-3FAs at doses about 5 or more times the standard dietary intake may yield antidepressant and/or mood-stabilizing effects. Most studies have used EPA monotherapy or a combination of EPA and DHA; few studies have examined DHA alone. Various reviews and meta-analyses of depression studies with n-3 fatty acids[15,16,17,18,19] generally support the efficacy of n-3FAs, but are limited by mixed studies of augmentation and monotherapy, small sample sizes, inclusion of bipolar subjects, different preparations of n-3FAs with varied ratios of EPA/DHA, and doses ranging from 1 to 10 g/d. A few representative studies are highlighted here.

EPA and EPA/DHA Combinations for Unipolar Major Depressive Disorder

Peet and Horrobin[20] conducted a randomized, placebo-controlled, dose-finding study of ethyl-eicosapentaenoate (ethyl-EPA) as adjunctive therapy for 70 adults with unipolar major depressive disorder (MDD) who were not responsive to standard antidepressants. A dose of 1 g/d ethyl-EPA for 12 weeks yielded significantly higher response rates (53%) than placebo (29%), with notable improvement of depressed mood, anxiety, sleep disturbance, libido, and suicidality. The 2 g/d group showed no significant separation between drug and placebo, and the 4 g/d group showed a nonsignificant trend toward improvement. These results suggested a therapeutic window for n-3FA required for maximum benefit, and it is possible that an "overcorrection" of the n-6FA:n-3FA ratio with higher n-3FA doses may limit the antidepressant effect of ethyl-EPA.

Su and colleagues[21] conducted an 8-week, double-blind, randomized, placebo-controlled trial comparing adjunctive n-3 (6.6 g/d EPA + DHA) with placebo in 28 depressed patients. Patients in the n-3FA group had a significant decrease in Hamilton-D (HAM-D) depression scores compared with placebo. In 20 subjects with MDD on antidepressant medication, Nemets and colleagues[22] found a statistically significant benefit of 1 g/d adjunctive EPA and a clinically important difference in mean reduction on the 24-item HAM-D scores by the study end point after 4 weeks, compared with placebo (12.4 vs 1.6 points). Overall response rates were 60% for EPA and 10% for placebo.

Frangou and colleagues[23] randomized 75 depressed subjects in a double-blind trial to receive 1 g/d ethyl-EPA, 2 g/d ethyl-EPA, or placebo for 12 weeks. EPA outperformed placebo significantly at both ethyl-EPA doses, based on HAM-D scores; the higher dose of ethyl-EPA seemed to confer no added benefit in comparison with 1 g/d. A recent randomized controlled study examining EPA monotherapy for depression found an advantage for EPA compared with placebo, although the study was limited by a smaller than projected sample size.[24] A double-blind study was carried out by Grenyer and colleagues[25] with a sample of 83 depressed outpatients randomized to tuna fish oil or placebo in addition to conventional treatment for 4 months. Results suggested good compliance and robust improvement in depressive symptoms but no significant differences between treatment groups at any time point. In all the aforementioned studies, EPA was well tolerated.

DHA for Unipolar MDD

Marangell and colleagues[26] performed a 12-week placebo-controlled study with 36 subjects that showed lack of efficacy of DHA (2 g/d) monotherapy for depression. Response rates were 27.8% for DHA and 23.5% for placebo, although DHA showed a modest advantage in mean improvement in the HAM-D, Montgomery-Asberg Depression Rating Scale (MADRS), and Global Assessment of Functioning (GAF) scales. On the other hand, a double-blind 3-armed dose-finding study of DHA monotherapy[27] demonstrated greater efficacy for DHA doses of 1 g/d in comparison with 2 g/d and 4 g/d. A therapeutic window for DHA similar to that seen for EPA may exist.[20] The DHA dose-finding study was limited by the lack of a placebo arm. Nonetheless, these studies suggest that DHA may work better at lower doses, and there may be an "overcorrection effect" if n-3FAs are dosed too high.

A recent meta-analysis by Sublette and colleagues[19] found that EPA, rather than DHA, appeared to have the main antidepressant effect. Their conclusion was based on the fact that all the significant positive omega-3 studies on depression in their review had at least 60% EPA, whereas all studies with less than 60% EPA were negative. As it stands, the evidence as a whole is more supportive of EPA than of DHA, or at least formulations whereby the ratio of EPA to DHA is higher than 3:2.

Omega-3 Fatty Acids in Perinatal Depression

Freeman and colleagues[28] performed a double-blind dose-finding trial of omega-3 in 16 women with postpartum depression. Subjects received 0.5 g/d, 1.4 g/d, or 2.8 g/d. HAM-D and Edinburgh Post Natal Depression Scale scores both decreased by approximately 50% for all groups, and there seemed to be no dose-response effect. Marangell and colleagues[29] found no preventive effect for postpartum depression in an open study with 2960 mg/d of an EPA/DHA mix in a small sample of pregnant women. A more recent prospective large-scale study[30] found no association between fish intake or n-3FA intake and risk of postpartum depression. Various lines of investigation have demonstrated benefit from n-3FAs for expectant mothers, in whom fish intake is often restricted during pregnancy, and for unborn children and infants, particularly with regard to neural development[31,32] and allergy prevention.[33] In fact, many prenatal vitamins now include an n-3FA supplement.

To date there have been 3 placebo-controlled trials of n-3FAs for the treatment of perinatal depression. In one study, Su and colleagues[34] found a significant benefit of n-3FA for the treatment of depression during pregnancy; however, 2 other studies have not shown a benefit of n-3FA over placebo in pregnant and postpartum women with MDD.[35,36] Therefore, at present it is premature to recommend n-3FAs as a primary treatment for perinatal depression. Nevertheless, for many pregnant and postpartum women n-3FA supplementation may be a reasonable augmentation strategy, considering the benefits of n-3FAs for both maternal and infant health. Despite the apparent safety of n-3FAs, the safe upper limit of these supplements during pregnancy is not known.[32] Pregnant women who are depressed and are considering omega-3 therapy should therefore discuss the matter with their physician. Patients should use only products whose labels indicate that they are free from mercury, polychlorinated biphenyls, or other contaminants, though recent evidence suggests that capsules generally do not contain these. Moreover, n-3FAs should be refrigerated to prevent oils from becoming rancid.

Omega-3 Fatty Acids in Bipolar Disorder

In the first clinical trial of omega-3 for bipolar illness, Stoll and colleagues[37] administered high doses of an n-3FA mix (6.2 g/d EPA plus 3.4 g/d DHA) to 30 patients with bipolar disorder I or II in a comparison with placebo over a 4-month period. Kaplan-Meier survival analysis revealed a significantly longer duration of remission for those receiving the adjunctive n-3FA mix versus placebo along with their current mood-stabilizing regimen. However, Keck and colleagues[38] were unable to replicate these results in a larger-scale study. In their double-blind, placebo-controlled trial of adjunctive EPA, 6 g/d, for 4 months in patients who had bipolar depression (n = 57) or rapid cycling (n = 59), outcomes with EPA did not differ from those with placebo. It should be noted that the differences in outcomes could be due to patient selection and to the forms of n-3FAs administered. For instance, the bipolar-depression or rapid-cycling group may not respond as well as the bipolar I or II group based on the Kaplan-Meier curve. Rapid-cycling subjects would also be less likely to have a longer duration of remission. Finally, the first study used EPA plus DHA, whereas the second study used EPA only.

Osher and colleagues[39] found benefit in a small study of 12 bipolar I patients in the depressed phase of the illness. Patients received 1.5 to 2 g/d open adjunctive EPA for up to 6 months. Ten patients completed at least 1 month of follow-up, and 8 achieved a 50% or greater reduction in HAM-D scores. No cycling occurred with any patients. In a study of 75 patients with bipolar depression, Frangou and colleagues[23] compared ethyl-EPA at 1 g/d or 2 g/d, versus placebo for 12 weeks. EPA outperformed placebo significantly in both EPA treatment arms, based on HAM-D scores. Higher doses of EPA appeared to confer no added benefit compared with 1 g/d.

Sarris and colleagues[40] have performed a recent meta-analysis of 6 selected studies, with one analysis focusing on bipolar depression and the other on bipolar mania. With regard to bipolar depression the investigators observed a significant but moderate effect in favor of n-3FAs (Hedges g = 0.34; P = .029). In bipolar mania, there was a nonsignificant trend in favor of n-3FAs (Hedges g = 0.20; P = .099). These meta-analyses, as well as other systematic reviews, have suggested that most of the benefit in bipolar subjects is probably related to depressive rather than manic symptoms.[41,42,43] Finally, there is preliminary evidence that n-3FAs may reduce anger and irritability in bipolar disorder.[44,45]

OMEGA-3 FATTY ACIDS IN OTHER PSYCHIATRIC DISORDERS

In other psychiatric syndromes, n-3FAs have been studied to a lesser extent than in mood disorders. Conditions investigated in small studies include borderline personality disorder, schizophrenia, attention-deficit disorder (ADD), obsessive-compulsive disorder (OCD), and Tourette disorder. These investigations tend to consist of smaller patient samples, and their conflicting results reflect this limitation. Selected studies from this body of work are reviewed here.

Omega-3 Fatty Acids in Psychotic Disorders

Fenton and colleagues[46] compared EPA, 3 g/d with placebo in 87 subjects with schizophrenia and schizoaffective disorder. After 16 weeks of treatment, no significant advantage was found for EPA over placebo. Of note, subjects in this study had been ill for longer than in previous case reports and case series that had suggested potential benefits in psychotic disorders.

Peet and Horrobin[47] performed a 12-week multicenter dose-finding study comparing EPA (1, 2, and 4 g/d) with placebo in 115 subjects with schizophrenia. Doses of 2 g/d and 4 g/d decreased triglyceride levels in patients taking clozapine. Doses of 2 g/d improved scores on the Positive and Negative Syndrome Scale, but the high placebo response rate resulted in a nonsignificant difference compared with placebo. The clozapine-treated patients showed little placebo effect in comparison with the rest of the sample, and EPA had a significant effect on all outcome scales.

Omega-3 Fatty Acids in Borderline Personality Disorder

Zanarini and Frankenburg[48] compared EPA, 1 g/d versus placebo in 30 women with borderline personality disorder. EPA significantly outperformed placebo in reduction of aggressive and depressive symptoms, although improvement also occurred in the placebo group. EPA resulted in a drop from 22.7 to 7.2 in the Modified Overt Aggression Scale (MOAS) score, and a change from 17.7 to 6.2 in the MADRS score. Scores in the placebo group dropped from 27.6 to 12.9 in the MOAS and from 18.0 to 8.0 in the MADRS. Comparison between the two treatment groups showed a significant advantage for EPA over placebo on both outcome measures.

Omega-3 Fatty Acids for Obsessive-Compulsive Disorder

Fux and colleagues[49] performed a placebo-controlled crossover trial of adjunctive EPA for OCD in a sample of 11 patients with inadequate response to selective serotonin uptake inhibitors (SSRIs). Subjects remained on their SSRI and were randomized to 6 weeks of placebo followed by 6 weeks of EPA, 2 g/d, or vice versa. Outcome measures included the Yale-Brown Obsessive-Compulsive Scale (YBOCS), and the HAM-D and HAM-A scales. No treatment-related effects were observed, although YBOCS scores improved in both treatment arms. Because treatment of OCD with all psychotropics usually requires 9 to 12 weeks for improvement, the observed lack of response may be due to the short duration of the treatment period.

Omega-3 Fatty Acids and Self-Harm

In a 12-week randomized controlled trial by Hallahan and colleagues,[50] 49 patients presenting after acts of repeated self-harm were randomized to receive, in addition to standard psychiatric care, a combination of 1.2 g EPA + 0.9 g DHA or placebo. At 12 weeks, the n-3FA group had significantly greater improvements in scores for depression, suicidality, and daily stresses. Scores for impulsivity, aggression, and hostility did not differ between treatment arms.

Lewis and colleagues[51] published a case-control study of suicide deaths among active-duty military, in which higher serum DHA appeared to have a protective effect against suicide, whereas EPA conferred only a trend to significance regarding protective effects. This result was especially intriguing in view of the body of evidence that seemed to favor the antidepressant benefit of EPA over DHA in the meta-analysis by Sublette and colleagues[19] (discussed in Ref.[52]).

OMEGA-3 FATTY ACIDS IN PEDIATRIC POPULATIONS

n-3FAs may be especially well suited to pediatric populations, in that they are considered important in brain development (especially DHA). There are some preliminary data in mood and developmental disorders. An exhaustive discussion of the various pediatric studies is beyond the scope of this review, although a few key data are highlighted.

Omega-3 Fatty Acids for Developmental Disorders

A recent review and meta-analysis of n-3FA supplementation for children with symptoms of attention-deficit/hyperactivity disorder (ADHD)[53] examined 10 clinical trials with a total of 699 children. Results suggested a modest but significant benefit regarding ADHD symptoms, particularly when the supplement was rich in EPA. The investigators cautioned that n-3FAs overall did not have the same degree of benefit as registered pharmacotherapies, but suggested that n-3FAs might be useful as an adjunct to these agents, given their safety and tolerability coupled with modest efficacy. Other studies have examined n-3FA therapy for childhood aggression,[54] autism,[55] and Tourette disorder,[56] with generally modest or mixed results.

Omega-3 Fatty Acids for Childhood Mood Disorders

Nemets and colleagues[57] performed a 16-week double-blind randomized controlled trial with 26 children of ages 6 to 12 years. Subjects were randomized to an omega-3 mix or placebo. Significant improvements were found using the Children's Depression Rating Scale, Children's Depression Inventory, and Clinical Global Impression.

Wozniak and colleagues[58] performed an 8-week open-label study with 20 children aged 6 to 17 years with bipolar disorder. Monotherapy with 1290 mg to 4300 mg combined EPA and DHA yielded a significant but modest reduction of 8.9 ± 2.9 points on the Young Mania Rating Scale (YMRS). Only 35% had a response by the usual criteria of a greater than 50% decrease on the YMRS. A more recent study suggested possible benefit from flax oil (ALA) in pediatric bipolar disorder.[7]

Overall, the results in pediatric populations are encouraging but should be considered preliminary.

SAFETY AND TOLERABILITY

The omega-3s have been shown to be very safe and well tolerated. Most complaints of side effects, such as gastrointestinal upset and fishy aftertaste, tend to occur with higher doses (greater than 5 g/d) and with less pure preparations. At the more typical doses of 1 g/d with highly purified omega-3 preparations, these adverse effects are less common.[15] There has been some concern about the possibility of bleeding with doses greater than 3 g/d, although this risk seems to be minimal, except in patients who are taking other agents that also affect platelet function.

Rare cases of increased bleeding times have been reported in patients taking aspirin or anticoagulants together with n-3FAs,[59,60] and platelet-function effects from n-3FAs have been demonstrated.[61] Individuals with bleeding disorders or who are taking anticoagulants such as warfarin or aspirin need to be carefully monitored for changes in serum International Normalization Ratios under physician supervision,[15] which may alert the clinician to the risk of bleeding. Although the clinical trials of n-3FAs in bipolar samples have generally supported safety, there have been a few reported cases of cycling in bipolar patients,[15] although direct causation can be hard to prove. Considering this along with the more modest evidence as a monotherapy for bipolar disorder, n-3FAs should be used with care in this population, perhaps with a concomitant mood stabilizer.

RECOMMENDATIONS

Given the apparent safety and tolerability of n-3FAs, their psychotropic effectiveness, particularly in mood disorders, deserves continued investigation. The data supporting use of n-3FAs for depression are the most encouraging, especially with regard to EPA. Low doses of n-3FA appear to be an effective and well-tolerated monotherapy or adjunctive therapy for depressed adults, although most clinical trials thus far have used n-3FAs as adjunctive agents. A recent review by Freeman and colleagues[15] recommends that depressed individuals may safely use approximately 1 g/d of an EPA/DHA mixture but should not substitute n-3FAs for conventional antidepressants at present. Likewise, individuals who take more than 3 g/d of an omega-3 preparation should do so under a physician's supervision.[15] This warning may be especially relevant for bipolar populations, in whom higher doses (6–10 g/d) have been used and in whom there may be a risk of cycling.[15]

The n-3FAs may be particularly well suited for the treatment of specific patient populations for whom antidepressants must be used with caution.[62] Such patients may include pregnant or lactating women, elderly people who may not tolerate side effects of conventional antidepressants, and people with cardiovascular disease or autoimmune conditions for which there may be dual benefits. There is some evidence that n-3FAs may be better suited to cases of more severe MDD, but the results are heterogeneous.[62]

Despite the mostly encouraging data, the authors cannot yet say whether the n-3FAs (and which ones) are truly effective antidepressants and/or mood stabilizers. This statement is even more tentative for psychotic disorders, OCD, and ADD, which have much more limited data, most of which is not encouraging. Controlled trials of n-3FA monotherapy are still limited, as are comparisons against standard agents in depression and the other aforementioned psychiatric conditions. Likewise, the issue of whether EPA, DHA, or a combination of the two is more effective in the treatment of depression remains to be clarified. Finally, the mechanism of action of the n-3FAs, particularly their interplay with the immune system, merits further investigation. Findings are under analysis from a study recently completed at Massachusetts General Hospital and Emory University, addressing the comparative efficacy of EPA and/or DHA as well as the role of lipid levels and immune biomarkers as moderators and mediators of response. It is hoped that these and other future investigations will help to clarify some of the unanswered questions about this exciting and potentially valuable treatment.

APPENDIX: REFERENCES

The complete reference list is online at http://www.psych.theclinics.com/dx.doi.org/10.1016/j.psc.2012.12.002.

KEY REFERENCES

6. Stoll AL. Omega-3 fatty acids in mood disorders: a review of neurobiological and clinical actions. In: Mischoulon D, Rosenbaum J, editors. Natural medications for psychiatric disorders: considering the alternatives. Philadelphia: Lippincott Williams & Wilkins; 2008. p. 39–67.
15. Freeman MP, Hibbeln JR, Wisner KL, et al. Omega-3 fatty acids: evidence basis for treatment and future research in psychiatry. J Clin Psychiatr 2006;67:1954–67.
17. Lin PY, Su KP. A meta-analytic review of double-blind, placebo-controlled trials of antidepressant efficacy of omega-3 fatty acids. J Clin Psychiatry 2007;68(7):1056–61.
19. Sublette ME, Ellis SP, Geant AL, et al. Meta-analysis of the effects of eicosapentaenoic acid (EPA) in clinical trials in depression. J Clin Psychiatry 2011;72(12):1577–84.
31. Greenberg JA, Bell SJ, Ausdal WV. Omega-3 fatty acid supplementation during pregnancy. Rev Obstet Gynecol 2008;1(4):162–9.
40. Sarris J, Mischoulon D, Schweitzer I. Omega-3 for bipolar disorder: meta-analyses of use in mania and bipolar depression. J Clin Psychiatry 2012;73(1):81–6.
41. Parker G, Gibson NA, Brotchie H, et al. Omega-3 fatty acids and mood disorders. Am J Psychiatry 2006;163(6):969–78.
42. Montgomery P, Richardson AJ. Omega-3 fatty acids for bipolar disorder. Cochrane Database Syst Rev 2008;(2):CD005169.

53. Bloch MH, Qawasmi A. Omega-3 fatty acid supplementation for the treatment of children with attention-deficit/hyperactivity disorder symptomatology: systematic review and meta-analysis. J Am Acad Child Adolesc Psychiatry 2011;50(10): 991–1000.
62. Appleton KM, Rogers PJ, Ness AR. Updated systematic review and meta-analysis of the effects of n-3 long-chain polyunsaturated fatty acids on depressed mood. Am J Clin Nutr 2010;91(3):757–70.

Nutrients for Prevention and Treatment of Mental Health Disorders

Shahin Akhondzadeh, PhD, FBPharmacolS[a],*,
Patricia L. Gerbarg, MD[b], Richard P. Brown, MD[c]

KEYWORDS

- Vitamins • Minerals • N-Acetylcysteine • Choline • 5-Hydroxy-L-tryptophan
- γ-Aminobutyric acid • Inositol • Neuroprotection

KEY POINTS

- Vitamin B_6 (pyridoxine) can reduce medication-related extrapyramidal side effects.
- Vitamin D_3 (cholecalciferol) studies in depression show mixed results; however, patients with prior history of depression, adolescents with severe mental illness, and people with reduced sun exposure may benefit.
- Medication augmentation with zinc may be beneficial in depression and attention-deficit disorder, but not in dementia.
- In children with low levels of serum ferritin, supplementation may improve learning, memory, and symptoms of attention-deficit/hyperactivity disorder.
- N-Acetylcysteine is an effective treatment for acetaminophen poisoning, antidepressant augmentation, and reduction of negative symptoms, abnormal movements, and akathisia in schizophrenia.
- Citicoline (CDP-choline) is beneficial in dementia, recovery from head injury, and probably acute ischemic stroke.
- Although studies supporting the use of inositol are small, evidence indicates benefits in depression, panic disorder, obsessive-compulsive disorder, bipolar depression, grooming disorders, and eating disorders.

Disclosures: None.
[a] Psychiatric Research Center, Roozbeh Hospital, Tehran University of Medical Sciences, South Kargar Street, Tehran 13337, Iran; [b] New York Medical College, 86 Sherry Lane, Valhalla, NY 12401, USA; [c] Columbia University College of Physicians and Surgeons, 30 East End Avenue, New York, NY 10028, USA
* Corresponding author.
E-mail address: s.akhond@neda.net

Psychiatr Clin N Am 36 (2013) 25–36
http://dx.doi.org/10.1016/j.psc.2012.12.003
0193-953X/13/$ – see front matter © 2013 Elsevier Inc. All rights reserved.

INTRODUCTION

The nutrients most relevant to clinical psychiatric practice are those that affect the central nervous system (CNS) and that are most likely to fall below the levels required for healthy brain function.[1,2] Dietary deficiencies, malabsorption, stress, illness, aging, brain injury, and genetic polymorphisms affect requirements for essential nutrients. Under conditions of oxidative stress, hypoxia, inflammation, or mitochondrial insufficiency, greater amounts of nutrients may be necessary to maintain cellular function and repair, and to prevent cumulative damage. The clinical research and biochemistry of S-adenosylmethionine, folate, and vitamin B_{12} are discussed in the article Folate, B_{12}, SAM-e by Bottiglieri, and omega-3 fatty acids in the article Omega-3 Fatty Acids in Psychiatry by Mischoulon and Freeman, elsewhere in this issue.

VITAMINS B_1, B_6, AND D
Vitamin B_1: Thiamine

The discovery of Vitamin B_1 (thiamine) deficiency as the cause of beriberi and Wernicke-Korsakoff syndrome (dementia, confabulation) led to the routine use of intramuscular and oral thiamine supplementation in the treatment of alcoholism. Critically ill patients are also at risk for thiamine deficiency and can benefit from supplementation.

Vitamin B_6: Pyridoxine

A review of vitamin B_6 (pyridoxine) found a lack of evidence to support its use in the treatment of depression, except in premenopausal women.[3] Low levels of pyridoxyl 5′-phosphate (PLP), the active form of vitamin B_6, have been significantly associated with depressive symptoms, but causality has not been established. B_6 deficiency (serum PLP <20 ng/mL) doubled the likelihood of depression in a cross-sectional study of older adults.[4]

Reactive carbonyl compounds (RCOs) are thought to contribute to the pathogenesis of schizophrenia. Vitamin B_6 detoxifies RCOs. In a 26-week, double-blind, placebo-controlled (DBPC) crossover trial, 50 inpatients with schizophrenia or schizoaffective disorder and tardive dyskinesia (TD) were given either vitamin B_6 (1200 mg daily) or placebo. The mean decreases on the Extrapyramidal Symptom Rating Scale, parkinsonism subscale score, and dyskinesia subscale scores were significantly greater in patients taking vitamin B_6 than in controls.[5]

Vitamin D_3: Cholecalciferol

Vitamin D deficiency during brain development has been linked to autism spectrum disorders and schizophrenia. In preclinical studies vitamin D deficiency affected differentiation of neurons, connectivity, dopamine pathways, and brain function. Evidence also suggests that vitamin D affects neurotransmitters, inflammatory markers, homeostasis of brain calcium, hypothalamic-pituitary-adrenocortical axis response to threat, and synthesis of nerve growth factor.[6] Adult population studies indicate that suboptimal vitamin D levels may increase risks for depression, Alzheimer's disease (AD), Parkinson's disease, and cognitive decline.[7] Although controversial, Vitamin D status is usually based on serum concentrations of 25-hydroxyvitamin D (25(OH)D): deficiency at less than 20 ng/mL; insufficiency at 20 to 30 ng/mL; and optimal at 30 to 80 ng/mL.

A review of 42 case-control, cohort, and randomized trials found a prevalence of vitamin D insufficiency in 40% to 100% of community-dwelling adults aged 65 years or older.[8] Among 104 adolescents seeking treatment for serious acute mental illness, vitamin D deficiency was found in 34% and insufficiency in 38%, with a strong association between vitamin D deficiency and psychotic features.[9]

Small clinical trials show positive effects of vitamin D on symptoms of depression. However, larger-scale epidemiological studies report mixed results. The heterogeneity of findings may be explained by differences in test measures, population characteristics, vitamin D doses, and study duration. For example, a cross-sectional study of 12,594 adults at a primary care clinic found that higher levels of vitamin D were associated with significantly reduced risk of depression. Individuals with a prior history of depression showed a strong correlation compared with no significant correlation in those without a prior history of depression.[6] Studies not taking this distinction into account might produce less valid results. Higher dietary intake of vitamin D correlated with a reduced risk of AD over 7 years in 480 community-dwelling women aged 75 years and older. The risk of other dementias showed no significant association.[10] Methodological weaknesses included the use of self-administered food-frequency questionnaires and lack of serum 25(OH)D measurements.

Current evidence is not sufficient to justify vitamin D supplementation in all depressed individuals. Assessment of 25(OH)D levels and supplementation with vitamin D may be indicated in patients with the following risks: older than 65 years; prior history of depression; adolescents with severe mental illness; lifestyle without regular outdoor activity; and residence in northern latitudes. In patients with documented insufficiency of vitamin D, a daily dose of 800,000 IU/d vitamin D_3 (cholecalciferol) for several weeks is recommended.[11] Once serum levels return to normal, a lower maintenance dose of 2000 to 6000 IU/d is usually adequate. Small trials of vitamin D for seasonal affective disorder have produced mixed results.[12,13]

MINERALS: ZINC, IRON, COPPER
Zinc

Zinc is important for immune regulation, energy metabolism, sexual function, insulin storage, and macromolecule stabilization; and modulation of protein synthesis, DNA transcription,[14] neuronal precursor cell activity, neurotrophins, neurotransmitters, and antioxidants.[15]

Major depression

Evidence from animal and human studies suggests an association between zinc status and mood disorders. A systematic review[16] identified 4 eligible randomized controlled trials (RCTs) of moderate quality. In 2 studies antidepressant augmentation with zinc (7–25 mg/d) for 10 to 12 weeks significantly improved depressive symptoms in comparison with placebo add-on. However, evidence for efficacy of zinc monotherapy was insufficient. The third RCT of 674 Guatemalan elementary school children (no DSM-IV diagnosis) at risk for zinc deficiency found no effect of zinc supplementation on mental health. However, increases in serum zinc concentrations were associated with decreases in internalizing symptoms (depression and anxiety). The fourth study found weak evidence of beneficial effects of zinc on mood in nondepressed subjects.[17]

Dementia

In healthy states zinc, copper, and amyloid-β (Aβ) metabolism are in a fine balance. Zinc may protect against Aβ-mediated oxidative cytotoxicity. Paradoxically, accumulation of either zinc or Aβ could lead to zinc-induced and/or Aβ-mediated oxidative and cytotoxic damage.[18] Histopathological and case-control studies show increased levels of brain zinc, mostly in parietal lobes,[19] and reduced levels of serum zinc in patients with AD.[20] In a systematic review of 55 studies, no conclusive evidence for any effect of zinc on AD was found.[20]

Mental health in children

An 8-week double-blind randomized controlled trial (DBRCT) of low-birth-weight infants in Brazil found no significant impact on mental or psychomotor development with zinc 1 mg or 5 mg/d, or placebo at age 6 and 12 months. However, by year 1, infants given zinc 5 mg/d had the highest ratings on behavioral assessment.[21] A combination of iron 20 mg/d and zinc 20 mg/d for 6 months may improve motor development and exploratory behavior in infants at risk for micronutrient deficiency.[22] Several RCTs found no effect of zinc alone or in combination with iron on cognitive performance in children.

Zinc plays a role in attention-deficit/hyperactivity disorder (ADHD), possibly through modulation of neurotransmitters (particularly dopamine and norepinephrine), prostaglandins, and fatty acids.[23] Two of 3 RCTs reported that zinc modestly reduced hyperactivity and impulsivity, but not attention. The first compared 6 weeks of zinc sulfate (15–150 mg/d) monotherapy (n = 400) with placebo.[24] The second compared 12 weeks of zinc augmentation of methylphenidate (n = 44) with placebo add-on.[25] A third study in 52 children showed no effect of zinc glycinate (15 or 30 mg/d) after 8 weeks either alone or with methylphenidate on symptoms of ADHD, although zinc 30 mg/d lowered the required dose of methylphenidate by 37%.[26] Tolerability of zinc was comparable with placebo in all 3 studies.

Sexual dysfunction

Zinc is important for gonadal and sexual function. A systematic review of 4 parallel trials in patients with uremia and sexual dysfunction surmised that zinc supplementation significantly increased testosterone levels but had inconsistent, nonsignificant effects on libido and nocturnal penile tumescence.[27]

Wilson disease

Wilson disease (WD) is a genetic disorder characterized by hepatic and neuropsychiatric symptoms caused by excess deposition of copper. A systematic review, including 1 RCT and 12 heterogeneous observational studies, concluded that in general chelating agents were the most effective treatment. By contrast, zinc therapy was favored for presymptomatic patients and neurological symptoms because it had better tolerability and equal efficacy in these conditions.[28] In a retrospective study of 288 patients (median follow-up of 17.1 years), zinc therapy was associated with significantly more hepatic treatment failure and less transplantation-free survival in comparison with chelation. Patients with inadequate response to zinc generally responded better to chelating agents.[29]

Zinc toxicity

Zinc is generally well tolerated. At toxic levels zinc can interfere with copper metabolism, causing symptoms of copper deficiency such as microcytic anemia and neutropenia. Acute zinc intoxication can also cause gastrointestinal disturbances, tachycardia, shock, and damage to pancreas and liver. Toxic doses exceed 150 mg/kg body weight, which is considerably more than clinical doses.[14]

Clinical guidelines

Based on the studies reviewed, the following guidelines are suggested:

1. Zinc supplementation of antidepressants might be beneficial in the treatment of depression.
2. Zinc alone or in combination with stimulants might improve hyperactivity and impulsivity symptoms of ADHD.

3. Zinc is a good choice for treatment of presymptomatic WD as well as its neurological symptoms.
4. Zinc is not beneficial for the treatment of dementia.
5. Zinc has minimal impact on intelligence quotient or mental health in children, except possibly in those with zinc deficiency.

Iron

Iron is essential for energy production, DNA and neurotransmitter synthesis, myelination, and phospholipid metabolism. Iron deficiency has been linked to movement disorders, including restless leg syndrome (RLS), possibly attributable to effects on dopamine synthesis. The diagnosis of iron-deficiency RLS is easily missed, particularly in children with ADHD in whom leg movements may be misinterpreted as a sign of hyperactivity. Iron deficiency is more common in children with ADHD. One study documented low levels of serum ferritin (a measure of iron stores) in 84% of 53 children with ADHD compared with 18% of 27 children who did not have ADHD. Lower ferritin levels correlated with more severe cognitive deficits and ADHD ratings.[30]

Studies of iron supplementation for the treatment of RLS have shown mixed results, which may be due to lack of measurement of serum ferritin levels, differences in populations studied, poor gastrointestinal absorption or brain uptake of supplements, genetic polymorphisms, or other dietary factors. A study of intravenous ferric carboxymaltose showed significant benefits in adults with RLS and low levels of ferritin.[31] In adolescents with iron deficiency, iron supplements improved learning and memory.[32] In a controlled study of 23 children (age 5–8 years) with low levels of serum ferritin, iron supplementation (80 mg/d) reduced ADHD symptoms.[33] Iron therapy was well tolerated. Larger studies are needed to explore the role of iron supplements in the treatment of ADHD.

Copper

Copper is essential in the synthesis of dopamine and norepinephrine. A Canadian study found that about 23% of children with ADHD were deficient in copper.[34] The role of copper in ADHD needs further study.

AMINO ACIDS, PRECURSORS, AND METABOLITES: *N*-ACETYLCYSTEINE, CHOLINE, L-TRYPTOPHAN, γ-AMINOBUTYRIC ACID, INOSITOL
N-Acetylcysteine

N-Acetylcysteine (NAC) is a precursor to the essential amino acid, cysteine. Unlike cysteine, NAC can penetrate the blood-brain barrier such that by oral supplementation, it can increase blood and brain levels of cysteine. Preclinical data, case reports, and clinical studies indicate potential benefits of NAC for the treatment of addictions, bipolar depression, schizophrenia, autism, obsessive-compulsive disorder (OCD), trichotillomania, nail biting, skin picking, overdoses, and environmental toxic exposures.[35]

NAC plays important roles in metabolic pathways believed to contribute to psychiatric disorders:

1. By increasing levels of brain cysteine, NAC was able to modulate glutamatergic and dopaminergic pathways. In vitro studies show a reduction in synaptic release of glutamate and an increase in dopamine release.[35]
2. Oxidative stress has been implicated as contributing to psychiatric disorders. Glutathione (GSH) is the body's main endogenous antioxidant. As a precursor to

GSH, NAC has been widely used to replenish GSH, for example in the treatment of acetaminophen overdose. In addition, NAC directly scavenges reactive oxygen species.

3. Inflammatory cytokines play a role in brain aging and psychiatric disorders. NAC has anti-inflammatory effects that may occur via antioxidant activities or other direct effects on inflammatory pathways.

Substance abuse

In an open-label study, 24 cannabis-dependent adults given NAC (2400 mg/d) showed no significant change in levels of urine cannabinoid. Nevertheless, scores on the Marijuana Craving Questionnaire improved.[36] In an 8-week DBRPC study, 116 cannabis-dependent adolescents were given NAC (1200 mg twice a day) as adjunct to contingency management and brief weekly cessation counseling. Compared with placebo, subjects taking NAC had more than twice the odds of negative urine tests.[37] In a 4-week open pilot study of 23 cocaine-dependent patients, higher doses of NAC (2400 mg/d or 3600 mg/d) improved retention rates compared with lower doses.[38] A small RCT of heavy smokers given NAC for 3 and a half days showed no statistically significant change in craving compared with placebo, but revealed a trend toward fewer withdrawal symptoms and reduced pleasure in smoking after abstinence.[39]

Obsessive-compulsive disorder, trichotillomania, nail biting, skin picking

In OCD, glutamatergic dysfunction has been implicated and glutamate modulating agents may be efficacious. It is postulated that NAC, by increasing extracellular glutamate concentration in the nucleus accumbens, could exert a therapeutic effect on OCD. Isolated case reports describe a significant response to NAC in patients with OCD and related grooming disorders.[35,40] One DBRPC trial of NAC for 50 patients with trichotillomania tested NAC 1200 mg/d for 6 weeks followed by NAC 2400 mg/d for 6 weeks more. Those given NAC showed reduced hair-pulling symptoms (P = .001) in comparison with placebo.[41]

Bipolar disorder

Increased oxidative stress has been associated with manic states and illness duration in bipolar disorder. Hyperdopaminergic states have been reported during mania. Both the antioxidant and dopaminergic modulatory effects of NAC might be beneficial in stabilizing patients with bipolar disorder. A 6-month DBRPC study of 75 patients with bipolar disorder demonstrated that NAC (2000 mg/d) as adjunct to established medication regimens resulted in significantly large improvements in depressive symptoms and global function when compared with placebo.[42]

Schizophrenia

Neurotransmitter abnormalities identified in schizophrenia patients include increased dopaminergic metabolism in the striatum, hypodopaminergia in the prefrontal cortex, and decreased glutamate levels in the prefrontal cortex. Oxidative stress has been associated with symptom severity, alterations in lipid membranes, mitochondrial dysfunction, and abnormalities in DNA, proteins, and dendritic sprouting.[35] In a 6-month DBRPC study of NAC (1000 mg twice a day) as adjunctive treatment to ongoing standard medications in 140 treatment-refractory schizophrenic patients with an average duration of symptoms of 12 years or more, those given NAC showed significant improvements in negative symptoms, global function, abnormal movements, and akathisia in comparison with placebo. Qualitative data revealed that patients in the NAC group achieved greater improvements in insight, self-care, social interaction, motivation, volition, psychomotor stability, mood stability, and auditory sensory processing.[43] NAC is a promising adjunctive treatment for schizophrenia and for reducing the side effects of psychotropic medications, particularly akathisia.

Detoxification following overdose or environmental exposures

Intravenous or oral NAC has been used for decades to treat acetaminophen poisoning. Acetaminophen is oxidized to *N*-acetyl-*p*-benzoquinoneimine (NAPQI), which binds to molecules inside hepatocytes, causing apoptosis and eventual hepatic necrosis. Glutathione (GSH) detoxifies NAPQI.[44] The depletion of GSH by acetaminophen toxicity can be reversed by NAC, leading to recovery and prevention of further damage. In addition to hepatoprotective properties, NAC is known to be renoprotective. It has been used to treat nephropathy caused by contrast injections during radiological studies. Considering its renoprotective effects and its benefits for bipolar disorder, it would be worth studying the use of NAC in preventing or treating renal dysfunction secondary to lithium treatment.

Side effects and adverse reactions

At clinically relevant doses, side effects of NAC are infrequent and generally mild. Occasionally allergic reactions and rarely anaphylactic reactions to intravenous NAC have been reported, but these rarely led to discontinuation. Longer-term and dose-finding studies would help clarify the maximum safe doses. In animal studies very high doses caused pulmonary hypertension, but this has not been reported in human studies. Overdose of NAC was associated with seizures. However, in low doses NAC is antiepileptic.

Tryptophan: 5-Hydroxy-L-Tryptophan

5-Hydroxy-L-tryptophan (5-HTP) is the immediate precursor of serotonin (5-hydroxytryptamine; 5-HT). Supplemental 5-HTP is used by many consumers for depression, insomnia, and fibromyalgia. 5-HTP replaced L-tryptophan, which was taken off the market in 1989 when a contaminated product from one manufacturer was associated with eosinophilia malignant syndrome. The absence of toxicity in 5-HTP has been documented in extensive studies.[45]

A review of 27 studies of 5-HTP for depression found that of the 11 DBRPC trials, 7 reported superiority over placebo, but only 5 of these showed statistical significance.[46] Studies have shown that 5-HTP augments the response to prescription antidepressants such as nialamide, clomipramine, and nomifensine. The average dosage of 5-HTP in adults is 200 to 300 mg/d in divided doses taken twice or 3 times per day. Limited evidence supports the use of 5-HTP as augmentation to antidepressant medications.

Common side effects of 5-HTP include nausea, vomiting, and diarrhea; less frequent are headache and insomnia. In rodents, doses below 50 mg/kg/d produce no toxicity, but doses above 100 mg/kg/d induce serotonin syndrome. There are no case reports of serotonin syndrome in humans taking 5-HTP alone or in combination with selective serotonin reuptake inhibitors. Studies report no adverse effects from a combination of 5-HTP and monoamine oxidase inhibitors.

γ-Aminobutyric Acid

γ-Aminobutyric acid (GABA) is the major inhibitory neurotransmitter in the brain. GABA inhibitory pathways help modulate overactivity of the amygdala, for example in anxiety disorders and posttraumatic stress disorder. It also has a regulatory role in cardiovascular, pituitary, renal, and immune function, as well as fertilization. In Japan, GABA is produced by fermentation and is used as a food supplement.

In a DBPC crossover study of 13 healthy adults, the effects on the electroencephalogram (EEG) of 100 mg GABA (Pharma-GABA) were compared with the effects of 200 mg L-theanine or placebo. GABA intake resulted in a significantly greater increase in alpha waves (associated with relaxed alertness) and decrease in beta waves (associated with high stress and difficulty concentrating) in comparison with L-theanine or placebo.[47] Low levels of salivary immunoglobulin A (IgA) occurring in highly anxious individuals decrease further under stress. In a DBRPC study, 8 patients with acrophobia (fear of heights) walked across a suspension bridge 54 m above the ground and 300 m long. In the placebo group, IgA levels (marker of stress and immune response) dropped substantially halfway across and at the end of the bridge. In the group given 100 mg GABA, IgA levels dropped only slightly midway and rose above baseline by the end of the bridge. GABA prevented decline in IgA, indicating reduced anxiety and stress effects.[47]

A synthetic analogue of GABA, pregabalin, approved by the US Food and Drug Administration for the treatment of neuropathic pain and partial-onset seizures, is being considered for approval as an adjunctive treatment for generalized anxiety disorder (GAD). Several RCTs confirm that in moderate to severe GAD, the anxiolytic effect of pregabalin is comparable with that of lorazepam (Ativan), alprazolam (Xanax), and venlafaxine (Effexor). Pregabalin is generally safe and well tolerated. Side effects include dizziness, somnolence, cognitive interference, incoordination, and headache. Drawbacks are the potential for some dependence and the slow onset of anxiolytic effect, which requires 1 week of daily treatment.[48] Starting with 50 mg 3 times daily, doses can be increased as tolerated.

Choline and its Precursors

Acetylcholine is derived from choline and acetyl coenzyme A. Neurons cannot synthesize choline and therefore must obtain it from the bloodstream following food absorption.[49,50] Dysfunction in cholinergic neurotransmission in the hippocampus and cortex is associated with dementia, particularly AD. Agents are being studied that could increase central cholinergic activity and thereby improve brain function in AD, other dementias, cerebrovascular accident, and other brain disorders.[51]

Trials of choline chloride (up to 200 mg/kg/24 h) failed to enhance acetylcholine biosynthesis or improve symptoms in patients with mild to moderate AD despite increasing levels of plasma choline.[52–54] Other supplements tested for the treatment of dementia by potentially increasing acetylcholine content and release include lecithin, cytidine 5'-diphosphocholine (CDP-choline), choline alphoscerate, and phosphatidylserine.[50] In a systematic review of 12 randomized studies, no study showed significant objective benefit of lecithin for AD or dementia of Parkinson's disease. Only 1 trial reported significant improvement following lecithin administration for subjective memory problems.[55]

Five trials of phosphatidylserine (average dose 300 mg/d) reported a modest benefit over placebo in the treatment of AD.[56–60] The effect of phosphatidylserine appears to be short term in light of the long-term disease progression.[60] Phosphatidylserine demonstrates mixed results in studies of age-associated cognitive impairment in non-demented individuals.[61–63] Differences in outcomes may be attributed to variations in study design, subject selection, duration, assessment instruments, and preparations of phosphatidylserine. A safety study reported no negative effects using 100 mg/d phosphatidylserine for 30 weeks.[64]

A review of 13 trials (total of 4054 patients), including 10 of patients with dementias, concluded that choline alphoscerate showed higher efficacy than placebo for cognitive symptoms and higher or similar efficacy in comparison with active treatment. Three other uncontrolled studies suggested that it might improve functional recovery in patients with acute cerebrovascular accident.[65] Results of a later open-label study noted improvement of cognitive function in Parkinson's dementia (n = 60) when compared with piracetam.[66]

CDP-choline (citicoline), a widely studied choline precursor, has been comprehensively reviewed.[67] A Cochrane systematic review of 14 studies with up to 12 months of follow-up concluded that CDP-choline improved memory and behavior, but showed no beneficial effect for attention.[68] Studies have demonstrated that citicoline can lead to resolution of brain edema, restoration of consciousness, and improvement in survival. Several trials have consistently demonstrated a beneficial role of citicoline (usual doses of 500–2000 mg/d) in prevention of head-injury sequelae,[67] including faster recovery of consciousness and memory function, accelerated resolution of neuropsychological disorders, shorter hospital stays, and improved EEG, quality of life, and motor recovery. Of importance, citicoline (intraperitoneal, intravenous, intramuscular, or oral) was tolerated well. Meta-analysis of 10 studies of cerebrovascular accidents (total of 2279 patients) concluded that receiving citicoline was associated with reduced morbidity and mortality.[69] Two drug-surveillance studies in more than 4300 patients with acute ischemic stroke showed that administration of oral citicoline (500–4000 mg/d) was associated with better outcomes, with no safety concerns.[70,71] Despite the previous reports on the benefit of citicoline in acute stroke, a recent multicenter DBRCT conducted in 2298 patients with moderate to severe acute ischemic stroke in 49 centers of 3 European countries did not provide any evidence for the superior effect of citicoline (1000 mg every 12 hours for 6 weeks) over placebo in global recovery.[72] There could be several reasons for these discrepant findings. Doses of 2000 mg/d were used in the study by Davalos and colleagues,[72] whereas the authors' clinical experience and the previous studies suggest better response to doses above 2000 mg/d. Furthermore, the effect of CDP-choline becomes evident usually after 9 to 12 weeks, whereas in the study by Davalos the duration was 6 weeks. In subgroup analysis, however, Davalos found evidence for the efficacy of citicoline in older patients (>70 years), in those with moderate stroke severity, and in patients not treated with a fibrinolytic. There is also some evidence for the role of citicoline in the treatment of cocaine addiction. In a 12-week RCT of 44 patients with a history of bipolar disorder and cocaine dependence, citicoline improved scores on the Rey Auditory Verbal Learning Test alternative word list (but not mood status) and reduced the probability of cocaine-positive urine significantly more than the placebo.[73] Not all studies, however, showed a beneficial effect on drug addiction.[67,74]

Picamilon

Picamilon, a cerebral vasodilator, is a composite of GABA and vitamin B_3 (niacin) that increases cerebral blood flow by reducing blood-vessel tone.[75] Most picamilon research is published in Slavic languages. This paragraph is based on abstracts, one review in English,[76] and clinical experience. In animal studies, picamilon is reported to exert mild tranquilizing action (reduced aggressive behavior) and mild stimulative activity that can improve alertness and cognitive function. It showed low toxicity (median lethal oral dose ≥ 10 g/kg of body weight). Additional controlled trials are indicated. In practice the authors (R.P.B. and P.G.) find that for patients with cerebral vascular impairment, picamilon can substantially improve alertness, confusion, anxiety, and depression. Side effects are mild, with occasional decreases in blood pressure.

Inositol

Inositol (cyclohexane-1,2,3,4,5,6-hexol), a carbohydrate, is a precursor of phosphatylinositol, a component of neuronal membranes, essential for effective signaling in adrenergic, cholinergic, serotonergic, and glutaminergic pathways. Although sometimes listed as a B vitamin, inositol is not a vitamin because it can be synthesized by the body. Several studies, including RCTs, show benefits greater than placebo in individuals with depression, panic, and OCD. A 1-month crossover DBRCT in 20 patients with panic disorder found similar improvements with inositol (18,000 mg/d) and fluvoxamine (up to 150 mg/d). However, inositol had fewer side effects.[77] Another DBRPC crossover study of 24 nondepressed patients with bulimia nervosa or binge-eating disorder compared inositol (18,000 mg) with placebo over 6 weeks. No other psychotropic medications were administered. In 5 patients side effects (mild abdominal pain, flatulence, or soft stools) remitted on reducing inositol to 12,000 mg/d. Compared with placebo, inositol significantly improved Global Clinical Impression and Visual Analog Scale scores, as well as showing a borderline significant effect on the Eating Disorders Inventory. Benefits were independent of anxiety or depression.[78]

In a DBRPC pilot study of 24 adults with bipolar depression (21 with bipolar I and 3 with bipolar II) whose mood stabilizers (lithium, valproate, and carbamazepine) were maintained, those given inositol (12,000 mg/d) augmentation showed greater improvement in depression ratings than those given placebo.[79] Another RCT of mood-stabilizer augmentation in 66 bipolar I patients and 11 patients with treatment-resistant depression demonstrated a recovery rate of 23.8% with lamotrigine versus 17.4% with inositol.[80] Although inositol can cause gastrointestinal side effects, particularly flatulence, it would be worth considering in bipolar patients requiring augmentation who experience side effects or lack of response with lamotrigine.

Although studies of inositol to date are few, evidence supports the use of this natural phospholipid precursor as an adjunctive treatment for depression, panic, OCD, bipolar depression, binge eating, and bulimia nervosa.

SUMMARY

Vitamins, minerals, and natural metabolites are essential for physical and mental health. In certain populations, such as children, those with ADHD, the elderly, patients with serious psychiatric or medical conditions, and substance abusers, vitamin deficiencies are not uncommon. For example, vitamin B_1 supplementation can reverse neurological symptoms in critically ill patients and in those with alcoholism. NAC and vitamin B_6 exemplify nutrients that are crucial for normal metabolism as well as for cellular protection and repair. By repairing neurological damage from antipsychotics and other psychotropics, NAC and B_6 can alleviate movement disorders and akathisia. Considerable evidence supports the use of citicoline (CDP-choline) in dementia, recovery from head injury, and probably acute ischemic stroke. Picamilon is a potentially useful vasodilator for the treatment of cerebrovascular insufficiency. Studies suggest that inositol can be beneficial in depression, panic disorder, OCD, bipolar depression, and eating disorders. Clinicians may opt to include nutrients in treatments offered to patients whose symptoms are not fully responsive to medications or in whom medications cause adverse effects.

APPENDIX: REFERENCES

The complete reference list is online at http://www.psych.theclinics.com/dx.doi.org/10.1016/j.psc.2012.12.003.

KEY REFERENCES

1. Brown RP, Gerbarg PL, Muskin PR. How to use herbs, nutrients, and yoga in mental health care. New York: W. W. Norton & Company; 2009.
5. Lerner V, Miodownik C, Kaptsan A, et al. Vitamin B6 treatment for tardive dyskinesia: a randomized, double-blind, placebo-controlled, crossover study. J Clin Psychiatry 2007;68(11):1648–54.
8. Barnard K, Colon-Emeric C. Extraskeletal effects of vitamin D in older adults: cardiovascular disease, mortality, mood, and cognition. Am J Geriatr Pharmacother 2010;8(1):4–33.
9. Gracious BL, Finucane TL, Freidman-Campbell M, et al. Vitamin D deficiency and psychotic features in mentally ill adolescents: a cross-sectional study. BMC Psychiatry 2012;12(1):38.
10. Annweiler C, Rolland Y, Schott AM, et al. Higher vitamin D dietary intake is associated with lower risk of Alzheimer's disease: a 7-year follow-up. J Gerontol A Biol Sci Med Sci 2012;67(11):1205–11.
16. Lai J, Moxey A, Nowak G, et al. The efficacy of zinc supplementation in depression: systematic review of randomised controlled trials. J Affect Disord 2012; 136(1–2):e31–9.
19. Schrag M, Mueller C, Oyoyo U, et al. Iron, zinc and copper in the Alzheimer's disease brain: a quantitative meta-analysis. Some insight on the influence of citation bias on scientific opinion. Prog Neurobiol 2011;94(3):296–306.
25. Akhondzadeh S, Mohammadi MR, Khademi M. Zinc sulfate as an adjunct to methylphenidate for the treatment of attention deficit hyperactivity disorder in children: a double blind and randomized trial [ISRCTN64132371]. BMC Psychiatry 2004;4:9.
26. Arnold LE, Disilvestro RA, Bozzolo D, et al. Zinc for attention-deficit/hyperactivity disorder: placebo-controlled double-blind pilot trial alone and combined with amphetamine. J Child Adolesc Psychopharmacol 2011;21(1):1–19.
33. Konofal E, Lecendreux M, Deron J, et al. Effects of iron supplementation on attention deficit hyperactivity disorder in children. Pediatr Neurol 2008;38(1):20–6.
35. Dean O, Giorlando F, Berk M. N-acetylcysteine in psychiatry: current therapeutic evidence and potential mechanisms of action. J Psychiatry Neurosci 2011;36(2): 78–86.
37. Gray KM, Carpenter MJ, Baker NL, et al. A double-blind randomized controlled trial of N-acetylcysteine in cannabis-dependent adolescents. Am J Psychiatry 2012;169(8):805–12.
39. Schmaal L, Berk L, Hulstijn KP, et al. Efficacy of N-acetylcysteine in the treatment of nicotine dependence: a double-blind placebo-controlled pilot study. Eur Addict Res 2011;17(4):211–6.
41. Grant JE, Odlaug BL, Kim SW. N-acetylcysteine, a glutamate modulator, in the treatment of trichotillomania: a double-blind, placebo-controlled study. Arch Gen Psychiatry 2009;66(7):756–63.
42. Berk M, Copolov DL, Dean O, et al. N-acetyl cysteine for depressive symptoms in bipolar disorder—a double-blind randomized placebo-controlled trial. Biol Psychiatry 2008;64(6):468–75.
43. Berk M, Copolov D, Dean O, et al. N-acetyl cysteine as a glutathione precursor for schizophrenia—a double-blind, randomized, placebo-controlled trial. Biol Psychiatry 2008;64(5):361–8.
44. Heard K, Green J. Acetylcysteine therapy for acetaminophen poisoning. Curr Pharm Biotechnol 2012;13(10):1917–23.

48. Bandelow B, Wedekind D, Leon T. Pregabalin for the treatment of generalized anxiety disorder: a novel pharmacologic intervention. Expert Rev Neurother 2007;7(7):769–81.
51. Brown RP, Gerbarg PL. Complementary and integrative treatments in brain injury. In: Silver JM, McAllister TW, Yudofsky SC, editors. Textbook of traumatic brain injury. 2nd edition. Washington, DC: American Psychiatric Press, Inc; 2011. p. 599–622.
67. Secades JJ. Citicoline: pharmacological and clinical review, 2010 update. Rev Neurol 2011;52(Suppl 2):S1–62 [in English, Spanish].
68. Fioravanti M, Yanagi M. Cytidinediphosphocholine (CDP-choline) for cognitive and behavioural disturbances associated with chronic cerebral disorders in the elderly. Cochrane Database Syst Rev 2005;(2):CD000269.
69. Saver JL. Citicoline: update on a promising and widely available agent for neuroprotection and neurorepair. Rev Neurol Dis 2008;5(4):167–77.
72. Davalos A, Alvarez-Sabin J, Castillo J, et al. Citicoline in the treatment of acute ischaemic stroke: an international, randomised, multicentre, placebo-controlled study (ICTUS trial). Lancet 2012;380(9839):349–57.
77. Palatnik A, Frolov K, Fux M, et al. Double-blind, controlled, crossover trial of inositol versus fluvoxamine for the treatment of panic disorder. J Clin Psychopharmacol 2001;21(3):335–9.
78. Gelber D, Levine J, Belmaker RH. Effect of inositol on bulimia nervosa and binge eating. Int J Eat Disord 2001;29(3):345–8.
80. Nierenberg AA, Ostacher MJ, Calabrese JR, et al. Treatment-resistant bipolar depression: a STEP-BD equipoise randomized effectiveness trial of antidepressant augmentation with lamotrigine, inositol, or risperidone. Am J Psychiatry 2006;163(2):210–6.

Phytomedicines for Prevention and Treatment of Mental Health Disorders

Patricia L. Gerberg, MD[a],*, Richard P. Brown, MD[b]

KEYWORDS

- Herbal • Adaptogens • *Rhodiola rosea* • Maca • Nootropics • Fatigue • Anxiety
- Cognitive function

KEY POINTS

- Many herb-drug interactions (HDIs) reported in preclinical, in vitro, and animal trials did not occur in human studies.
- Ginseng augments the activating effects of other agents, improving alertness, mental focus, energy, and cognitive function.
- In stable patients with schizophrenia, American ginseng (*Panax quinquefolius*) may improve verbal memory and reduce medication-related extrapyramidal symptoms.
- Balanced combinations of nootropics, herbs, and nutrients can improve anxiety, depression, memory, cognitive function and sexual function more than monotherapies.

INTRODUCTION

Phytomedicinal (herbal) compounds have a myriad of biological actions relevant to psychiatry: synthesis of neurotransmitters and their metabolizing enzymes, binding to neurotransmitters and receptors, membrane transport, stimulation or inhibition of central nervous system (CNS) activities, modulation of neuroendocrine systems, neuroprotection, enhancement of mitochondrial energy production, cellular repair, regulation of gene expression, and neurogenesis.[1,2]

The effects of most herbal medicines cannot be determined by analyzing individual constituents or by in vitro studies. In their excellent review, Sarris and colleagues[3] note that whole plant extracts can contain many bioactive compounds with synergistic and/or polyvalent effects. Synergy occurs when the sum of compounds exerting one main biologic effect is greater than their individual effects. Polyvalence refers to multiple biologic actions contributing to an overall effect when

---

Disclosure: None.
[a] New York Medical College, 40 Sunshine Cottage Road, Valhalla, NY 10595, USA; [b] Columbia University College of Physicians and Surgeons, 630 W 168th Street, New York, NY 10032, USA
* Corresponding author. 86 Sherry Lane, Kingston, New York.
E-mail address: PGerbarg@aol.com

Psychiatr Clin N Am 36 (2013) 37–47
http://dx.doi.org/10.1016/j.psc.2012.12.004
psych.theclinics.com

constituents have various physiologic effects or when one constituent has multiple effects. In addition, one constituent may affect absorption, distribution, metabolism, or excretion of other components. Furthermore, biochemical actions observed in vitro do not necessarily occur when herbs are consumed, digested, and metabolized in living organisms.

Purity and quality varies among products because of differences in root stock, soil, climate, harvest time, adulterants, and methods of extraction and drying. Resources that help identify high-quality brands[4] are available through the American Botanical Council (herbalgram.org) and fda.gov/medwatch, supplementwatch.com, ConsumerLab.com, and Drugs.com.

The selection of medicinal herbs for this article was based on credible clinical evidence of safety and efficacy, known biochemical mechanisms of action, usefulness in psychiatric practice, and the clinical experience of the authors. For research, phytochemistry, and genomics of *Rhodiola rosea, Eleutherococcus senticosus*, and *Schizandra chinensis*, see the article by Panossian; for *Ginkgo biloba*, the article by Diamond; for *St. John's wort*, the article by Sarris; and for *saffron, passion flower, valerian*, and *sage*, see the article by Ackhondzadeh in this issue.

HERB-DRUG INTERACTIONS

HDIs may enhance or interfere with therapeutic effects. Few herbs relevant to psychiatric practice have clinically significant medication interactions. Understanding the basic principles for evaluating herbs enables clinicians to safely use herbs to complement standard treatments while minimizing the risks of adverse events.

Pharmacokinetic and Pharmacodynamic Interactions

Pharmacokinetic interactions that affect medication serum levels most commonly include the induction or inhibition of cytochrome P450 (CYP450) isozymes and permeability glycoproteins (P-gp). Pharmacodynamic interactions involve risks of CNS side effects, hepatotoxicity, or bleeding. Additive effects can occur when an herb and a drug have similar effects, for example, if both are sedating, such that even though there are no pharmacodynamic interactions, the combination may cause excess sedation. Kennedy and Seely[5] reviewed studies of whole herb extracts from 21 herbs with evidence of HDIs in humans. Studies of single constituents were excluded because the concentration of an isolated constituent greatly exceeds that of the whole herb extract. The reviewers concluded that for most herbs with evidence of drug interactions in preclinical studies the effect on medication serum levels in humans is small and of no clinical significance. However, caution is required when combining herbs that interact with drugs having a narrow therapeutic window (a small difference between therapeutic and toxic levels or between therapeutic and subtherapeutic levels) and serious adverse effects outside the therapeutic range, for example, warfarin or digoxin. In addition, little clinical evidence exists regarding interactions of herbs with many anesthetics and antidepressants.

Minimizing Risks

The risks of HDIs can be minimized by monitoring for side effects and obtaining serum levels of medications that have a narrow therapeutic window. The vast majority of the alterations in drug levels involving herbs covered in this volume do not reach a level of clinical significance. Among herbs used in psychiatric practice, St. John's wort (*Hypericum perforatum*) has the greatest number of studies and reports showing interactions with drugs. See the discussion of *St. John's wort HDIs* in the article by *Sarris* in this issue and the review by Zhou and Lai.[6]

Herbal effects on CYP P450 isoenzymes in vitro and in many animal studies are often not found to occur in human studies. Oral ingestion, digestion, and metabolism alter bioactive compounds such that they may have no effect or even the opposite effect observed in vitro. Some constituents cancel the effects of others. In addition, the impact of a botanical extract on P450 metabolism of one drug does not necessarily generalize to other drugs metabolized by the same isoenzyme because herbs and drugs compete for binding to an isoenzyme. Different drugs have different affinities for an isoenzyme that may be stronger or weaker than the affinity of the herb.

Evidence of effects on three P-gp substrates (saquinavir, metronidazole, and talinolol) is available for *G. biloba*. Although digoxin is also a P-gp substrate, there is no evidence that the herbs discussed in this article affect digoxin levels.[5] Nevertheless, the authors advise measurement of digoxin levels after initiating or changing the dose of any herbal preparation known to induce P-gp. Certain herbs, particularly *Panax ginseng*, American ginseng, and *E. senticosus* produce false-positive results of modest interference with serum digoxin levels. This occurs because they can directly affect certain digoxin assays using fluorescence polarization immunoassay. However, ginsengs and Eleuthero do not interfere with enzyme-linked chemiluminescent, immunosorbent, and turbidimetric digoxin assays.[7]

Most HDI studies include only healthy subjects. Izzo and Ernst[8] reviewed 128 case reports and 80 clinical trials of HDIs for 7 herbs, including ginkgo, Asian ginseng, kava, and St. John's wort. Yap and colleagues[9] reviewed HDIs for anticancer drugs. *Herbal Contraindications and Drug Interactions* by Brinker[10] is a well-documented resource. Other compendia of natural treatments are useful for general information but often present data from poorly documented, inconclusive cases without adequate qualifications. Therefore, readers are advised to check individual citations on HDIs before drawing conclusions.

HERBAL MEDICINES FOR ANXIETY AND INSOMNIA

Two systematic reviews found evidence for herbal supplements containing chamomile (*Matricaria recutita*) or kava (*Piper methysticum*) in the treatment of anxiety.[3,11] Anxiolytic phytomedicines usually work via gamma-aminobutyric acid (GABA), the primary inhibitory neurotransmitter in the brain. Increasing GABAergic action reduces CNS stimulation and amygdalar overactivity (as occurs in anxiety disorders) (see the article by *Muench* in this issue).

Chamomile (M. recutita)

Although chamomile is widely used for anxiety and insomnia, research on this herb is limited. In a study of rat brain homogenates, chamomile extracts significantly inhibited GABA-metabolizing enzymes.[12] One component of chamomile, apigenin, has high affinity for benzodiazepine GABA receptors, modulates monoamine neurotransmission, and has neuroendocrine activity but causes minimal sedation. An 8-week randomized controlled trial (RCT) of moderately anxious patients with generalized anxiety disorder found that chamomile extract (220–1100 mg/d) significantly improved Hamilton Anxiety scores versus placebo.[13] Because the effects are mild, it is often necessary to combine chamomile with other sedative or anxiolytic herbs. Although generally low in side effects, as a member of the ragweed family, it can trigger allergic reactions.

Kava (P. methysticum)

Kava extract, a traditional ceremonial drink in South Pacific islands, contains active constituents, alpha-pyrones (kavalactones). Its actions include increased GABA transmission, blocking of lipid membrane sodium and calcium channels, monoamine oxidase B inhibition, and noradrenalin and dopamine reuptake inhibition. Kava has modest benefits in short-term studies of mild anxiety. Seven double-blind randomized placebo-controlled (DBRPC) studies (total $n = 380$) indicate significant improvement in HAMA scores with kava versus placebo.[14] Effect sizes were small, and only minor side effects were reported. Common side effects include gastrointestinal effect, allergic reactions, fatigue, headache, and light sensitivity; less common are restlessness, drowsiness, and tremor. Long-term heavy usage can lead to facial swelling, scaly rash, dyspnea, low albumin levels, increased gamma-glutamyl transferase (GGT) levels, decreased white blood cell and platelet counts, hematuria, and pulmonary hypertension.[15]

Case reports of kava hepatotoxicity, including 11 possible cases of liver failure, led to US Food and Drug Administration (FDA) warnings of potential liver injury.[16] Investigations implicate the use of incorrect plant parts or species, acetonic or ethanolic extraction, and inadequate storage resulting in hepatotoxic mold.[17] Ingestion of kava with alcohol, sedatives, or muscle relaxants can induce coma. In vitro studies found that kava extract and kava lactones inhibit P450 isoenzymes, CYP3A4, CYP2D6, and others involved in the metabolism of pharmaceuticals.[18] Sarris and colleagues[3] concluded that evidence supports the use of kava for anxiety but that safety issues need to be addressed. They recommend using only products from peeled roots of noble cultivars (species traditionally considered safe and therapeutic). Individuals with hepatic insufficiency should avoid kava. Monitoring liver functions in long-term users should be considered. There is no evidence to date regarding safety in children. Weighing mild benefits against risks of intoxication, abuse, dependency, medication interactions, and rare severe adverse reactions, the authors do not recommend kava until more information on safety, efficacy, quality, and reliable batch testing is available.

Theanine (Camellia sinensis)

Theanine is an amino acid found in *C. sinensis*, the herb in green tea, used for centuries for calming and medicinal effects. About 3 to 4 cups of green tea contain 60 to 160 mg of theanine. RCTs show some evidence of a mild relaxing effect, possible by inhibition of cortical excitation.[19,20] Theanine also has antioxidant and antiproliferative activities. In clinical practice, the authors use decaffeinated green tea for mild to moderate anxiety, particularly in patients who are sensitive to side effects from stronger agents. It has minimal and usually no side effects when started at 200 mg 1 to 3 times a day and titrated up to a maximum of 6 times a day. High doses can cause overactivation in patients with brain damage.

HERBAL ADAPTOGENS FOR ENERGY, MENTAL FOCUS, COGNITIVE ENHANCEMENT, AND SEXUAL FUNCTION

Herbal adaptogens contain hundreds of bioactive compounds, including metabolic regulators, and have demonstrated abilities to protect living organisms from damage caused by oxidative stress, toxic chemicals, infection, neoplasm, heat, cold, radiation, hypoxia, physical exertion, and psychological stress. See the article in this issue by *Panossian* for an in-depth discussion of research and mechanisms of action for important adaptogens, *R. rosea, E. senticosus*, and *S. chinensis*.

Korean or Asian Ginseng (Panax ginseng), American Ginseng (Panax Quinquefolius)

Ginsengs contain numerous bioactive compounds, particularly ginsenocides or ginseng saponins. *P. ginseng* increases nitric oxide production in endothelial cells, which is essential for blood flow and oxygen delivery. In a DBRPC 8-week study of healthy volunteers (older than 40 years) those given 400 mg/d ginseng had significantly better abstract thinking and reaction time compared with placebo. In a DBRPC crossover study of 32 healthy adults aged 18 to 40 years, 100 mg of *P. ginseng* significantly improved reaction time, accuracy, calmness, and working memory.[21] Average doses range between 300 and 800 mg/d. Side effects include over stimulation, anxiety, insomnia, tachycardia, gastrointestinal disturbance, headache, and reduced platelet aggregation. Use of anticoagulants is a contraindication.

American ginseng (*P. quinquefolius*) is less activating than Asian ginseng. In a 4-week DBRPC study of 64 stable patients with schizophrenia, those given American ginseng (preparation HT100) showed significant improvements in verbal memory and reduction in extrapyramidal symptoms compared with those given placebo.[22] In practice, ginsengs augment the activating effects of other agents, improving alertness, mental focus, energy, and cognitive function. American ginseng can reduce the anticoagulant effects of warfarin. In treating cognitive dysfunction due to stroke, trauma, or vascular disease, the authors get better results by combining *P. ginseng, P. quinquefolius*, and *E. senticosus*.

Maca (Lepidium Myenii)

Maca, a Peruvian herb that grows at high altitudes in the Andes, is used to enhance sexual function, fertility, energy, alertness, mental focus, mood, and physical resilience. Research on maca consists primarily of animal studies and a small number of methodologically limited human trials. For a review of published and unpublished studies see Gonzales.[23] Although studies suggested improvements in sexual desire and function, maca did not increase serum testosterone, luteinizing hormone, follicle-stimulating hormone, prolactin, or estradiol in men. In animal studies, the black variety of maca had positive effects on learning and memory, as well as decreasing acetylcholinesterase (AChE) levels in ovariectomized mice. In vitro studies found that maca reduced human brain malondialdehyde levels (marker of oxidative stress). A DBRPC pilot study found that maca (3.0 g/d) significantly reduced selective serotonin reuptake inhibitor–induced sexual dysfunction.[24] Toxic effects have not been reported in animal or human studies using herb that has been boiled before consumption. Animal studies found no teratogenic or carcinogenic effects. A population study comparing Peruvians living at high altitude who regularly consumed maca (starting with maca juices in childhood) with those living at lower altitudes who did not consume maca found that the maca users had better overall health and lower systolic blood pressure, body mass index, and rate of bone fractures. In recommended doses, maca causes minimal side effects; excess doses may cause overactivation. In clinical practice, the authors find that maca can be a useful adjunctive treatment for neural fatigue, sexual dysfunction, and infertility.

Arctic Root (R. rosea)—Clinical Guidelines

R. rosea can be beneficial in many conditions: fatigue from any cause; cognitive dysfunction; memory problems; depression; stress-related conditions; sexual dysfunction; weakness; infection; and cancer.[4,25] See article by *Panossian* in this issue for research review and mechanisms of action. When given alone or in combination with other adaptogens, it can enhance physical and intellectual performance, attention, and memory. *R. rosea* absorbs best when taken on an empty stomach 20 minutes before breakfast and 20 minutes before lunch. Capsules may contain 100 to 180 mg dry root extract. The usual starting dose is 1 capsule before breakfast, increasing by 1 capsule every 3 to 7 days as needed. For patients who are sensitive to stimulants, prone to anxiety, elderly, or medically ill, starting with a fraction of a capsule reduces the risk of overstimulation. It is possible to open a capsule, dissolve the contents in juice or tea, store in an 8-ounce refrigerated container and titrate smaller amounts gradually. The average adult doses range is 150 to 600 mg/d, although some people respond to 25 mg/d.

As with other adaptogens, *R. rosea* may be taken before and during a stressful period or continuously long-term for chronic conditions. In some cases, the beneficial effects may fade after a few weeks or months. If this occurs, the dose could be increased, if necessary, up to a maximum tolerable dose (600–900 mg/d). Should this fail to restore efficacy, then "holidays"—discontinuation for 1 to 3 weeks at a time—may be indicated. Patients usually report improved energy during the first week on adequate doses. If this does not occur, or if efficacy fades, it is important to check the *R. rosea* brand to be certain it is of high quality.

Side effects

R. rosea is considered to be safe; adverse effects are rare. In some cases of individual sensitivity, anxiety, irritability, insomnia, headache, and rarely palpitations may occur. *R. rosea* stimulative effects can exacerbate agitation and irritability in bipolar disorder, although it can ameliorate depressive episodes in patients taking mood stabilizers. During the first 2 weeks, some patients report vivid dreams but not nightmares. If taken in the late afternoon or evening, stimulative effects can disturb sleep. Some individuals report increased libido and occasionally hypersexuality. Unlike amphetamines, *R. rosea* does not cause addiction or withdrawal symptoms. The onset of action is gradual and lasts 4 to 6 hours. At doses more than 600 mg/d, *R. rosea* can reduce platelet aggregation, resulting in increased bruising in some patients. No cases of bleeding have been attributed to *R. rosea*. It is advisable to monitor and adjust doses of anticoagulant medication and to discontinue aspirin and other substances that could affect bleeding. The herb should be discontinued 1 week before surgery. Although *R. rosea* showed in vitro inhibitory effects on CYP isoenzymes, in vivo rat studies found no significant effects on CYP450 metabolism of theophylline or warfarin or on anticoagulant activity of warfarin.[26]

In clinical practice, *R. rosea* can reduce menopause-related symptoms of fatigue, impaired cognitive function and memory, depression, and loss of libido. Anecdotally, in menopausal women who are amenorrheic for less than 12 months, resumption of menses while taking this adaptogen has been observed occasionally. Animal studies suggest that *R. rosea* binds to estrogen receptors but does not activate them.[4] In vitro *R. rosea* did not increase proliferation of human breast cancer cells.[4]

S. chinensis—Clinical Guidelines

S. chinensis is useful as an adjunctive treatment for sluggish depression, chronic fatigue, and fibromyalgia. It has been studied in combination with *R. rosea* and *E. senticosus* (see review by Panossian).[27] In vitro *S. chinensis* inhibited CYP3A4 enzymes. Paradoxically, in vivo animal studies showed it induces the same isozymes. In animal models, schisandra reduced warfarin levels, but this has not been demonstrated in humans. Until more is known, international normalized ratio (INR) should be monitored in patients on anticoagulants who are given schisandra.[28]

HERBAL COGNITIVE ENHANCERS

Herbal cognitive enhancers, called nootropics, have been widely used in Europe and Asia for centuries, yet they are virtually unknown to most American physicians. Generally low in side effects, nootropics have shown significant benefits in the treatment of cerebral ischemia, stroke, vascular dementia, hypoxic ischemia due to birth trauma, traumatic brain injury, age-related memory decline, and schizophrenia.[4]

Vinpocetine (Vinca minor)

Derived from periwinkle (*Vinca minor*) leaves, vinpocetine, a cerebral vasodilator, inhibits Ca^{2+}calcium/calmodulin-dependent cyclic guanosine monophosphate (cGMP) phosphodiesterase and increases intracellular cGMP in cerebral vascular smooth muscle, leading to decreased resistance, vasodilation, and increased flow in cerebral blood vessels. It also inhibits platelet aggregation and increases erythrocyte deformability, reducing blood viscosity and further enhancing blood flow.[28,29] Cerebral vasodilation, antioxidant, and antiinflammatory activities support the use of vinpocetine for ischemic stroke and other brain injuries. Most clinical studies of vinpocetine used small samples and short durations, limiting the conclusions that can be drawn. A photon emission tomographic (PET) study showed improved cerebral glucose kinetics and blood flow in peristroke areas.[30] In a 1-year study of 61 children with hypoxic ischemic encephalopathy from intracranial birth trauma, vinpocetine reduced seizure frequency, intracranial hypertension, and psychomotor sequelae.[31]

Vinpocetine has been shown to be safe, even in infants and the elderly, with only mild side effects of indigestion, nausea, headache, drowsiness, facial flushing, insomnia, headache, and dry mouth. Agranulocytosis was reported rarely. By selectively increasing cerebral, but not peripheral blood flow, vinpocetine is less likely to cause hypotension than other vasodilators, and it can be helpful in patients with magnetic resonance imaging, single-photon emission computed tomography, or PET scan evidence of blood flow abnormality.

Galantamine—Snowdrop (Galanthus nivalis)

In folk medicines of Russia and Europe, extract of snowdrop (*G. nivalis*) was used to prevent age-related memory decline. Galantamine (Razadyne), FDA approved for treatment of Alzheimer disease (AD), is a synthetic copy of 1 component of snowdrop. It is an allosteric modulator of nicotinic receptors and a weak inhibitor of AChE.[32,33] In an open trial, 280 patients with AD from the Swedish Alzheimer Treatment Study were given galantamine starting with 8 mg/d and gradually increasing to 24 mg/d as tolerated. After 3 years, rather than the expected decline, subjects had mean increases of 2.6 points on Mini Mental Status Examination (MMSE) and 5.6 points in Alzheimer Disease Assessment Scale-cognitive subscale.[34] For patients who do not tolerate gastrointestinal side effects of prescription galantamine, *G. nivalis* combined with *R. rosea* can be as effective and more tolerable.

Huperzine-A (Huperzia serrata)

Huperzine-A, an alkaloid derived from Chinese club moss (*H. serrata*) is a strong, selective, reversible AChE inhibitor with neuroprotective properties, including protection against free radicals, amyloid-β protein formation, glutamate, and ischemia.[35] It protects mitochondria, reduces oxidative stress, and upregulates nerve growth factor. Huperzine-A is rapidly absorbed, readily penetrates the blood-brain barrier, and has a long duration of AChE inhibitory action. In animal and primate studies, it improves learning and memory.[35,36] Three double-blind trials with more than 450 people and 1 open trial done in China showed significant benefits in AD. In a DBRPC study of 78 patients with mild to moderate vascular dementia, those given Huperzine-A, 0.1 mg twice a day, significantly improved in scores on the MMSE, clinical dementia rating, and activities of daily living (ADL) after 12 weeks (P<.01), with no significant adverse events.[37] A 16-week DBRPC study of 210 individuals with mild to moderate AD reported cognitive enhancement only at doses more than 0.4 mg/d at week 16.[38] Other trials showed positive outcomes in vascular dementia, traumatic brain injury, age-related memory decline, and schizophrenia.[39,40] Huperzine-A is well tolerated with few side effects and minimal peripheral cholinergic effects.

Centrophenoxine (Meclofenoxate, Lucidril)

Centrophenoxine (CPH) is an ester of dimethyl-aminoethanol (DMAE), a component in choline synthesis, and p-chlorophenoxyacetic acid, a synthetic form of a plant growth hormone.[41] Elevation of brain acetyl choline is one mechanism for therapeutic effects in cerebral atrophy, dementia, and TBI. CPH also delivers DMAE rapidly to the brain where it is incorporated into nerve cell membranes as phosphatidyl-DMAE, an avid scavenger of OH-radicals.[42] In rat models of cerebral ischemia, CPH reduced cognitive deficits, suggesting a preventive role in cerebrovascular disease.[43] The administration of CPH (100 mg/kg body weight/d, intraperitoneal) to aged rats for 6 weeks resulted in increased activity of catalase, superoxide dismutase, glutathione reductase, and glutathione in brain tissues. Lipid peroxidation significantly decreased.[44]

In an 8-week DBRPC trial in patients with moderate dementia CPH showed increased psychomotor and behavioral performance in about 50% of subjects compared with 27% on placebo.[45] A 3-month DBRPC study of 62 geriatric patients with mild to moderate AD found that those given antagonic stress (a preparation of CPH, vitamins, and nutrients) showed significant improvements in memory, cognitive function, and behavior compared with those given nicergoline. Data suggest that nootropics work better when combined with vitamins, minerals, and other nootropics, such as piracetam.[46,47]

SUMMARY AND FUTURE DIRECTIONS

Phytomedicines contain bioactive compounds that can alleviate neuropsychiatric symptoms when used alone or in combination with other herbs, nutrients, and psychotropic medications. Evidence for the beneficial effects of herbal extracts on oxidative stress, mitochondrial energy production, cellular repair, neurotransmission, CNS activation or inhibition, neuroendocrine systems, and gene expression is expanding. Understanding the psychopharmacology and the potential clinical effects on anxiety, insomnia, cognitive function, and sexual function enables clinicians to evaluate the supplements being taken by patients and to advise them on safety and efficacy. Advances in testing constituents of herbal extracts continue to improve assessment of supplement quality. "Herbomics" is the use of proteomic, genomic, and other "omic" technologies to investigate the effects of herbs on gene regulation.[3] These and other modern technologies are improving the identification of specific herbal constituents, their mechanisms of action, and new therapeutic applications. Genetic studies will help evaluate the purity of rootstocks, develop more potent subspecies with greater specificity and diversity of therapeutic effects, and the accurately monitor the quality of products.

REFERENCES

1. Brown RP, Gerbarg PL, Muskin PR. Alternative treatments in psychiatry. In: Tasman A, Kay J, Lieberman J, editors. Psychiatry. 3rd edition. London: John Wiley & Sons, ltd; 2008. p. 2318–53.
2. Brown RP, Gerbarg PL. Complementary and integrative treatments in brain injury. In: Silver JM, McAllister TW, Yudofsky SC, editors. Textbook of traumatic brain injury. 2nd edition. Washington, DC: American Psychiatric Press, Inc; 2011. p. 599–622.
3. Sarris J, Panossian A, Schweitzer I, et al. Herbal medicine for depression, anxiety and insomnia: a review of psychopharmacology and clinical evidence. Eur Neuropsychopharmacol 2011;21(12):841–60.
4. Brown RP, Gerbarg PL, Muskin PR. How to use herbs, nutrients, and yoga in mental health care. New York: W. W. Norton & Company; 2009.
5. Kennedy DA, Seely D. Clinically based evidence of drug-herb interactions: a systematic review. Expert Opin Drug Saf 2010;9(1):79–124.
6. Zhou SF, Lai X. An update on clinical drug interactions with the herbal antidepressant St. John's wort. Curr Drug Metab 2008;9(5):394–409.
7. Dasgupta A, Tso G, Wells A. Effect of Asian ginseng, Siberian ginseng, and Indian ayurvedic medicine Ashwagandha on serum digoxin measurement by Digoxin III, a new digoxin immunoassay. J Clin Lab Anal 2008;22(4):295–301.
8. Izzo AA, Ernst E. Interactions between herbal medicines and prescribed drugs: an updated systematic review. Drugs 2009;69(13):1777–98.
9. Yap KY, Kuo EY, Lee JJ, et al. An onco-informatics database for anticancer drug interactions with complementary and alternative medicines used in cancer treatment and supportive care: an overview of the OncoRx project. Support Care Cancer 2010;18(7):883–91.
10. Brinker F. Herbal contraindications and drug interactions plus herbal adjuncts with medicines. 4th edition. Sandy (OR): Eclectric Medical Publications; 2010.
11. Lakhan SE, Vieira KF. Nutritional and herbal supplements for anxiety and anxiety-related disorders: systematic review. Nutr J 2010;9:42.
12. Awad R, Levac D, Cybulska P, et al. Effects of traditionally used anxiolytic botanicals on enzymes of the gamma-aminobutyric acid (GABA) system. Can J Physiol Pharmacol 2007;85(9):933–42.
13. Amsterdam JD, Li Y, Soeller I, et al. A randomized, double-blind, placebo-controlled trial of oral *Matricaria recutita* (chamomile) extract therapy for generalized anxiety disorder. J Clin Psychopharmacol 2009;29(4):378–82.
14. Feucht C, Patel DR. Herbal medicines in pediatric neuropsychiatry. Pediatr Clin North Am 2011;58(1):33–54, x.
15. Mathews JD, Riley MD, Fejo L, et al. Effects of the heavy usage of kava on physical health: summary of a pilot survey in an aboriginal community. Med J Aust 1988;148(11):548–55.
16. U.S. Food and Drug Administration. Letter to health care professionals: FDA issues consumer advisory that Kava products may be associated with severe liver injury. 2002. Available at: http://www.fda.gov/Food/ResourcesForYou/Consumers/ucm085482.htm. Accessed October 25, 2011.
17. Teschke R, Sarris J, Lebot V. Kava hepatotoxicity solution: a six-point plan for new kava standardization. Phytomedicine 2011;18(2–3):96–103.
18. Mathews JM, Etheridge AS, Black SR. Inhibition of human cytochrome P450 activities by kava extract and kavalactones. Drug Metab Dispos 2002;30(11):1153–7.

19. Kimura K, Ozeki M, Juneja LR, et al. L-Theanine reduces psychological and physiological stress responses. Biol Psychol 2007;74(1):39–45.
20. Lu K, Gray MA, Oliver C, et al. The acute effects of L-theanine in comparison with alprazolam on anticipatory anxiety in humans. Hum Psychopharmacol 2004; 19(7):457–65.
21. Reay JL, Scholey AB, Kennedy DO. *Panax ginseng* (G115) improves aspects of working memory performance and subjective ratings of calmness in healthy young adults. Hum Psychopharmacol 2010;25(6):462–71.
22. Scholey A, Ossoukhova A, Owen L, et al. Effects of American ginseng (*Panax quinquefolius*) on neurocognitive function: an acute, randomised, double-blind, placebo-controlled crossover study. Psychopharmacology 2010;212(3): 345–56.
23. Gonzales GF. Ethnobiology and ethnopharmacology of *Lepidium meyenii* (maca), a plant from the Peruvian Highlands. Evid Based Complement Alternat Med 2012; 2012:193496.
24. Dording CM, Fisher L, Papakostas G, et al. A double-blind, randomized, pilot dose-finding study of maca root (*L. meyenii*) for the management of SSRI-induced sexual dysfunction. CNS Neurosci Ther 2008;14(3):182–91.
25. Brown RP, Gerbarg PL, Ramazanov Z. A phythomedical review of *Rhodiola rosea*. Herbalgram 2002;56:40–62.
26. Panossian A, Hovhannisyan A, Abrahamyan H, et al. Pharmacokinetic and pharmacodynamic study of interaction of *Rhodiola rosea* SHR-5 extract with warfarin and theophylline in rats. Phytother Res 2009;23(3):351–7.
27. Panossian A, Wikman G. Pharmacology of *Schisandra chinensis* Bail.: an overview of Russian research and uses in medicine. J Ethnopharmacol 2008; 118(2):183–212.
28. Wang BL, Hu JP, Sheng L, et al. Effects of *Schisandra chinensis* (Wuweizi) constituents on the activity of hepatic microsomal CYP450 isozymes in rats detected by using a cocktail probe substrates method. Yao Xue Xue Bao 2011; 46(8):922–7 [in Chinese].
29. Patyar S, Prakash A, Modi M, et al. Role of vinpocetine in cerebrovascular diseases. Pharmacol Rep 2011;63(3):618–28.
30. Szilagyi G, Nagy Z, Balkay L, et al. Effects of vinpocetine on the redistribution of cerebral blood flow and glucose metabolism in chronic ischemic stroke patients: a PET study. J Neurol Sci 2005;229–230:275–84.
31. Dutov AA, Gal'tvanitsa GA, Volkova VA, et al. Cavinton in the prevention of the convulsive syndrome in children after birth injury. Zh Nevropatol Psikhiatr Im S S Korsakova 1991;91(8):21–2 [in Russian].
32. Raskind MA, Peskind ER, Wessel T, et al. Galantamine in AD: a 6-month randomized, placebo-controlled trial with a 6-month extension. The Galantamine USA-1 Study Group. Neurology 2000;54(12):2261–8.
33. Tariot PN, Solomon PR, Morris JC, et al. A 5-month, randomized, placebo-controlled trial of galantamine in AD. The Galantamine USA-10 Study Group. Neurology 2000;54(12):2269–76.
34. Wallin AK, Wattmo C, Minthon L. Galantamine treatment in Alzheimer's disease: response and long-term outcome in a routine clinical setting. Neuropsychiatr Dis Treat 2011;7:565–76.
35. Zhao Y, Zhao B. Natural antioxidants in prevention and management of Alzheimer s disease. Front Biosci (Elite Ed) 2012;4:794–808.
36. Tang XC. Huperzine A (shuangyiping): a promising drug for Alzheimer's disease. Zhongguo Yao Li Xue Bao 1996;17(6):481–4.

37. Xu F, Hongbin H, Yan J, et al. Greatly improved neuroprotective efficiency of citicoline by stereotactic delivery in treatment of ischemic injury. Drug Deliv 2011; 18(7):461–7.
38. Rafii MS, Walsh S, Little JT, et al. A phase II trial of huperzine A in mild to moderate Alzheimer disease. Neurology 2011;76(16):1389–94.
39. Akhondzadeh S, Abbasi SH. Herbal medicine in the treatment of Alzheimer's disease. Am J Alzheimers Dis Other Demen 2006;21(2):113–8.
40. Wang R, Yan H, Tang XC. Progress in studies of huperzine A, a natural cholinesterase inhibitor from Chinese herbal medicine. Acta Pharmacol Sin 2006;27(1): 1–26.
41. Nandy K. Centrophenoxine: effects on aging mammalian brain. J Am Geriatr Soc 1978;26(2):74–81.
42. Nagy K, Dajko G, Uray I, et al. Comparative studies on the free radical scavenger properties of two nootropic drugs, CPH and BCE-001. Ann N Y Acad Sci 1994; 717:115–21.
43. Liao Y, Wang R, Tang XC. Centrophenoxine improves chronic cerebral ischemia induced cognitive deficit and neuronal degeneration in rats. Acta Pharmacol Sin 2004;25(12):1590–6.
44. Bhalla P, Nehru B. Modulatory effects of centrophenoxine on different regions of ageing rat brain. Exp Gerontol 2005;40(10):801–6.
45. Pek G, Fulop T, Zs-Nagy I. Gerontopsychological studies using NAI ('Nurnberger Alters-Inventar') on patients with organic psychosyndrome (DSM III, Category 1) treated with centrophenoxine in a double blind, comparative, randomized clinical trial. Arch Gerontol Geriatr 1989;9(1):17–30.
46. Schneider F, Popa R, Mihalas G, et al. Superiority of antagonic-stress composition versus nicergoline in gerontopsychiatry. Ann N Y Acad Sci 1994;717:332–42.
47. Fischer HD, Schmidt J, Wustmann C. On some mechanisms of antihypoxic actions of nootropic drugs. Biomed Biochim Acta 1984;43(4):541–3.

Adaptogens in Mental and Behavioral Disorders

Alexander G. Panossian, PhD, DSci

KEYWORDS

- ADAPT-232 • Adaptogen • Salidroside • Fatigue • Depression • Bipolar disorder
- Anxiety • Posttraumatic stress disorder

KEY POINTS

- Clinical efficacy and safety of the most extensively studied adaptogens, *Rhodiola rosea*, *Eleutherococcus senticosus* and *Schisandra chinensis* in mental and behavioral disorders, including stress induced fatigue, chronic fatigue, depression, neurosis, bipolar disorder and schizophrenia. Evidence for stress-protective and simulative effects.
- Recent studies on elucidation of molecular mechanisms. How adaptogens increase tolerance to stress? The effects on mediators of stress response, homeostasis, energy metabolism in the neuroendocrine-immune system on metabolic and transcriptional levels of regulation.

INTRODUCTION

The term adaptogen was introduced into scientific literature in 1958 to denote substances that increase the "state of nonspecific resistance" during stress, based on Hans Selye's theory of stress and the general adaptation syndrome.[1] Criteria for adaptogenic herbs include a high level of safety and normalization of body functions regardless of the nature of stressors.[2] In light of more recent research, adaptogens are redefined as "metabolic regulators which increase the ability of an organism to adapt to environmental stressors and prevent damage to the organism by such stressors."[3] Herbalists refer to adaptogens as rejuvenating herbs, qi tonics, rasayanas, or restoratives.[1] This article focuses on the most extensively studied adaptogens: *Rhodiola rosea*,[4] *Eleutherococcus senticosus*,[5] and *Schisandra chinensi*.[6] Clinical studies,[7,8] evidence for stress-protective and simulative effects,[1,9–11] molecular mechanisms of action on metabolic[12] and other processes regulated by the neuroendocrine system[13,14] are discussed. For clinical guidelines on safe and effective use of adaptogens, including herb-drug interactions, see the article Phytomedicines by Gerberg and Brown in this issue. Supplemental citations not listed in the References are available online at http://www.psych.theclinics.com.

Research and Development, Swedish Herbal Institute, Kovlingevagen 21, Vallberga, Halland 31250, Sweden
E-mail address: ap@shi.se

Psychiatr Clin N Am 36 (2013) 49–64
http://dx.doi.org/10.1016/j.psc.2012.12.005
0193-953X/13/$ – see front matter © 2013 Elsevier Inc. All rights reserved.

psych.theclinics.com

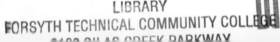

CLINICAL STUDIES

Starting in 1948, extensive research in the former Soviet Union found that adaptogens enhance physical and mental performance under stress.[1,6,15] They were beneficial in treating asthenodepressive syndrome and neurasthenia, conditions characterized by fatigue, weakness, irritability, headaches, malaise, insomnia, poor appetite, cognitive and memory impairments, stress, depression, and anxiety.[7–10,15] These symptoms are frequently observed following infectious and other illnesses or after intensive work requiring mental exertion. Interpretation of the studies before 1990 is limited by the heterogeneity of patient populations, outdated diagnostic nomenclature, and the mixed quality of methodology. Although most of the studies before 1990 would be rated as low quality by modern standards, they provide considerable information about efficacy and safety of adaptogens in the treatment of psychiatric disorders. Over the past 25 years, better quality studies have been published and reviewed.[1,2,5,7–10,15–29] **Tables 1** and **2** summarize a representative selection of older studies and all of the post-1985 studies relevant to mental health.

The systematic comparison of clinical trials of botanicals has an important limitation—herbal preparations are not absolutely identical, unlike synthetic psychotropics that are bioequivalent across studies. Chemical composition of herbal preparations depends on many factors, including

- Genetic factors
- Environmental factors
- Climate
- Soil characteristics (pH, fertilization, heavy metals)
- Infections (insects, pests, microbes)
- Parts of the plant used
- Processing (pulverization, extraction, solvent polarity, temperature, duration, distillation, expression, fermentation, purification)
- Storage (light, oxygen, humidity, temperature).

Comparison of standardized products with reproducible chemical composition best assures reproducible pharmacologic activity. The content of active markers in herbal products sold in health food stores can vary considerably.[75] Therefore, it is not surprising that clinical trials sometimes yield inconsistent outcomes for the same herb.

Rhodiola rosea L, Rhizome and Radix (Arctic Rhizome, Arctic Root)

For more than 60 years, clinical and biochemical studies of R rosea have increased our understanding of how this adaptogen exerts many of its therapeutic effects. The roots contain six groups of bioactive compounds, including phenylpropanoids, phenylethanol derivatives, flavonoids, monoterpenes, triterpenes, and phenolic acids. Rosavins, salidroside (rhodioloside), and tyrosol have been used as active marker compounds in standardized extracts. In 1969, the Pharmacologic Committee of the USSR Ministry of Health recommended the use of R rosea in patients suffering from asthenia neuroses, hypotension, and schizophrenia, as well as for healthy individuals doing intensive work, requiring mental or physical exertion.[15]

The dose-response curve of R rosea is bell shaped, decreasing at both low and high doses, such that maximal activity is at an intermediate dose. This optimal dose could be different for various R rosea preparations with different activity levels at the same dose.[4] In this context, the results obtained on Rhodiola SHR-5 extract in clinical trials cannot be extrapolated to other Rhodiola preparations produced by other manufacturers.

Table 1
Clinical trials of *E senticosus*, *R rosea*, and *S chinensis* in mental and behavioral disorders

Condition	Adaptogen	Design	Duration Weeks	Jadad Score	Number of Subjects	Level of Evidence	Reference
Bipolar disorder	E senticosus	R DBPC	6	5	76	1b	27
Chronic fatigue syndrome	E senticosus	RPCDB	4, 8, 16	5	96	1b	20
Fatigue syndrome (stress induced fatigue/burnout)	R rosea	RPCDB	4	5	60	Ib	25
Life-stress symptoms	R rosea	OL	4	1	101	IIa	19
Adults physical and cognitive deficiency	R rosea	OL	6, 12	0	120	III	35,a
Depression:							
	R rosea	RPCDB	6	5	91	Ib	17
	R rosea	OL, C^b	—	0	78/56^b	IIa	36,a
	E senticosus	OL, C^b	—	0	77	—	37,a
	S chinensis	OL, UC	—	0	37	—	38,a
Asthenodepressive syndrome (stress- induced depression)	R rosea	OL, UC	2-3	0	128	—	39,a
	R rosea	OL, UC	2-3	0	135/27	—	40,a
	R rosea	OL	8	0	58	—	41,a
	R rosea	OL	—	0	25	—	42,a
	S chinensis	OL, UC	—	0	13	—	43,a
	S chinensis	OL, UC	2-6	0	40	—	44,a
	S chinensis	OL	1.5	—	36	—	45,a
	S chinensis	OL	—	—	30	—	46,a
Neurosis (stress-induced depression)	R rosea	OL	1.5	0	65	—	47,a
	R rosea	PC, SB	—	1	70/80	—	48,a
	S chinensis	OL,	2-8	0	386^b	—	49,a
	S chinensis	OL	2-10	0	250	—	50,a
	E senticosus	OL, PC	3-4	2	80	—	51,52,66,67,a
Anxiety:	R rosea	OL	10	0	10	III	53,a
Schizophrenia	S chinensis	OL	—	0	79/41^b	III	54,55,a
	S chinensis	OL, C	—	0	30/20^b	—	48,a
	S chinensis	OL	—	0	48	—	56,a

Abbreviations: C, controlled; OL, open label trial; PC, placebo-controlled; R, randomized; SB, single blind; UC, uncontrolled.
a Citations not listed in the Key References are in Supplemental References 35–75 at http://www.psych.theclinics.com.
b Rating ranges from 1 to 5.
Data from Panossian A, Wikman G. Evidence-based efficacy of adaptogens in fatigue, and molecular mechanisms related to their stress-protective activity. Curr Clin Pharmacol 2009;4(3):198–219; and Panossian A, Wikman G. Effects of adaptogens on the central nervous system and the molecular mechanisms associated with their stress—protective activity. Pharmaceuticals 2010;3(1):188–224.

Table 2
Adaptogen effects on physical and mental fatigue in healthy adults under stress, results from selected clinical studies

Adaptogen Dose/Day Duration	Design[a]/Total Subjects	Primary Outcomes[b]	Quality of Evidence	Jadad Score[c]	Reference
R rosea SHR-5 (170 mg QD) vs placebo 2 wk	DBRPC, CO 2 parallel groups 56 healthy subjects[d] (24–35 y)	↓Mental fatigue, ↑perceptive and cognitive functions, associative thinking, short-term memory, calculation, concentration, speed of audio-visual perception.	Ib	4	2
R rosea SHR-5 (50 mg bid) vs placebo × 20 d	DBRPC 2 parallel groups 40 healthy (17–19 y)	↓Mental fatigue, ↑perceptive, well-being, ↑physical fitness, vs control (P<.01).	Ib	3	26
R rosea SHR-5 (single dose 370 mg or 555 mg) vs placebo	DBRPC 3 parallel groups 161 healthy, 20 untreated (19–21 y)	↑Capacity for mental work, ↑antifatigue vs control (P<.001); no significant difference between two dosage groups.	Ib	3	29
ADAPT-232 3 capsules acute	DBPC, CO 60 adults	↑Short-term memory, speed, reliability understanding information, precision in computer–based tests, ↓mistakes in psychometric tests	IIa	1	57,e
	DBPC, CO, 5 cosmonauts	↑Working capacity Russian cosmonauts during training 90-d isolation	IIa	1	58,e

Rhodosin (*R rosea*) 100 mg/20 d	DBPC 60	↑Physical fitness, ↓mental fatigue (*P*<.01) and ↑well-being (*P*<.05) vs control	IIa	1	59,e
Rodelim (*R rosea, E senticosus, S chinensis*) 100 mg/acute	DBPC 60	Rodelim improved mental working capacity in computer and correction tests against a background of fatigue.	IIa	1	60,e
ADAPT-232 Chisan	DBRPC 2 parallel groups 40 healthy subjects	Test of attention before and 2 h after ADAPT 270 mg: ↑mental speed & accuracy during mental fatigue vs placebo	Ib	5	16

[a] ↑, increase; ↓, decrease; CO, crossover; DB, double-blind; PC, placebo-controlled; R, randomized.

[b] According to WHO, FDA, and EMEA: Ia, meta-analyses of randomized and controlled studies; Ib, evidence from at least one randomized study with control; IIa, evidence from at least one well performed study with control group; IIb, evidence from at least one well performed quasiexperimental study; III, evidence from well performed nonexperimental descriptive studies as well as comparative studies, correlation studies, and case studies; and IV, evidence from expert committee reports or appraisals and/or clinical experiences by prominent authorities.

[c] Rating ranges from 1 to 5.

[d] Data not listed or unavailable.

[e] Citations not found in the Key References list are in Supplemental References 35–75 at http://www.psych.theclinics.com.

Data from Panossian A, Wikman G. Evidence-based efficacy of adaptogens in fatigue, and molecular mechanisms related to their stress-protective activity. Curr Clin Pharmacol 2009;4(3):198–219; and Panossian A, Wikman G. Effects of adaptogens on the central nervous system and the molecular mechanisms associated with their stress–protective activity. Pharmaceuticals 2010;3(1):188–224.

Fatigue

Numerous systematic reviews concluded that *R rosea* standardized extract SHR-5 is significantly beneficial in stress-induced fatigue.[7,8,21,23] In a double-blind, randomized, placebo-controlled (DBRPC) 4-week study of subjects with fatigue syndrome, *R rosea* significantly reduced fatigue and improved attention.[25] Moreover, in randomized controlled trials in healthy adults, *R rosea* (SHR-5) demonstrated antifatigue effects and improved cognitive functions during fatigue and under stressful conditions.[26,28,29]

Depression

A 6-week DBRPC study of *R rosea* (SHR-5) in mild-to-moderate depression showed significant antidepressant effect. Two groups were each given a different *R rosea* dose (340 mg/day and 680 mg/day); the third group received placebo. Both treatment groups showed significant improvements in depression on Hamilton Depression Scale (HAMD) and Beck Depression Index[3] compared with placebo. The herb also reduced insomnia, emotional instability, and somatization, as well as improving self-esteem. In subjects with a variety of depressive conditions being treated with tricyclic antidepressants, adjunctive *R rosea* reduced the time spent in hospital.[39,40] Addition of *R rosea* increased activity and intellectual and physical productivity, and decreased tricyclic-induced side effects.

Augmentation of medication benefits and reduction of medication side effects

R rosea was reported to alleviate psychotropic side effects in schizophrenic subjects.[39,40] This short communication noted that 31 subjects suffering from pronounced neuroleptic-induced extrapyramidal symptoms (EPS) received a high dose of *R rosea* (25–40 drops; 2–3 times daily) for 1 to 1.5 months. In addition, 19 of these subjects were given a combination of high dose *R rosea* and an anticholinesterase, trihexyphenidyl (Romparkin) (Trihexyphenidyl alone had failed to alleviate EPS.). *R rosea* had a pronounced therapeutic effect on neuroleptic-induced parkinsonian symptoms and fatigue.

Eleutherococcus senticosus, Acanthopanax senticosus (Eleuthero or Siberian Ginseng)

E senticosus, also called *Acanthopanax senticosus*, a thorny shrub that grows in Siberia and northern China, has been used in traditional herbal medicine for symptoms of asthenia such as fatigue and weakness.[2,5] Eleven clinical trials of the effects of *E senticosus* on mental performance have been reviewed.[7,8]

Neurosis

In a placebo-controlled 3-arm study, 80 (38 men and 42 women) 23- to 55-year-old subjects with a history of 1 to 5 years of neurosis were given *E senticosus* 120 mg twice a day (corresponding to 0.5 mL liquid extract twice a day), or 240 mg twice a day (1 mL of the liquid extract twice a day) or placebo for 3 to 4 weeks. Compared to placebo, both doses of herb significantly improved sleep, well-being, appetite, stamina, cognitive function, and mood, without side effects.[51,52] The lack of randomization and unclear diagnostic grouping limit the quality of this early study.

Chronic fatigue

Patients diagnosed as having idiopathic chronic fatigue, who were treated for 1 month with *E senticosus* root extract 2 g/day (about 9 mg of eleutherosides), significantly improved on Rand Vitality Index scores compared with placebo. A longer period of treatment for 2 months was less effective for the whole group but still significantly effective in a subset of subjects with mild-to-moderate fatigue.[20] These results indicate that in some patients with idiopathic chronic fatigue adaptogen effects may fade over time. In such cases, wash-out periods may be useful during long-term treatment. Similar results have been observed in some clinical studies of Rhodiola[28] and Schisandra.[61–63]

Bipolar disorder

The effectiveness of *E senticosus* (750 mg 3 times a day) compared with fluoxetine (20 mg am) as an adjunct to lithium (serum lithium levels 0.6–1.2 mmol/L) in Chinese adolescents with bipolar disorder was evaluated in a 6-week double-blind, randomized, controlled trial.[27] Outcomes were defined as follows:

- Response was improvement of greater than 50% on HAMD-17
- Remission was HAMD-17 less than 7
- Switching to mania was a score greater than 16 on the Young Mania Rating Scale and meeting criteria for mania based on the *Diagnostic and Statistical Manual of Mental Disorders.*

After 6 weeks of treatment, response and remission rates of the *E senticosus* group and the fluoxetine group were similar (67.6% vs 71.8%, and 51.4% vs 48.7%, respectively). There was a significant time effect ($F = 183.06$; $P<.01$) but not a significant group effect ($F = 0.99$) or group by duration of treatment interaction ($F = 0.779$). In this study, *E* senticosus as an adjunct to lithium in bipolar adolescents was as effective as fluoxetine. Both treatments were well tolerated, but E senticosus had a better safety profile with fewer adverse events (10.8%) than fluoxetine (30.9%). Moreover, three subjects given fluoxetine switched to mania compared with no subject in the *E senticosus* group.[27] The use of *E senticosus* as an adjunct to mood stabilizers in bipolar disorder warrants further study.

Schisandra chinensis (Schizandra)

Extracts of *S chinensis* fruits and seeds have been used to reduce symptoms of stress such as fatigue and weakness, to enhance physical performance, and to promote endurance. Schizandra preparations were intensively studied in subjects with mental and behavioral disorders in the USSR after World War II (see review of 13 studies by Panossian and Wikman, 2009, 2010.)[7,8] Although older studies used different diagnostic criteria, they reported interesting findings that warrant further study. Administration of Schizandra (fruit and seed tincture, 1:5, 90% ethanol) for 16 to 40 days produced central nervous system (CNS) stimulation in all of 40 subjects with asthenia and depression.[44] Twenty-two subjects showed increased energy and physical activity, improved mood, remission of fatigue, and normalization of sleep. A series of trials involving 60 subjects with mental disorders[54,64,65] reported that Schizandra eliminated catatonic stupor in 31 schizophrenics and promoted remission of hallucinations. Also, in bipolar psychosis (n = 9), Schizandra decreased depression but did not alleviate hypomanic symptoms. In alcoholics, Schizandra hastened resolution of alcoholic delirium. In schizophrenia (n = 41) and chronic alcoholism (n = 197),[66] subjects given Schizandra (5–25 drops) became calmer, more sociable, more willing to work, and had decreased emotional tension and anxiety, increased facial mimicry, and better mood. In schizophrenic subjects (n = 32), Schizandra also improved verbalization and associative processes.[56] Administration of Schizandra with apomorphine reduced addiction to the opiate.[65,66] Schizandra also ameliorated side effects of tranquilizers and antidepressants (eg, sibazon, amitriptyline, relanium). In 23 out of 39 subjects (53.5%), increasing amitriptyline from 50 to 75 mg/day resulted in headaches, dizziness, flaccidity, xerostomia (dry mouth), and bowel and urinary disorders. In contrast, in Schizandra-treated subjects whose amitriptyline was increased from 50 to 75 mg, similar side effects occurred in only 4 out of 172 subjects (1.9%). Coadministration of tranquilizers and Schizandra enabled the use of optimal doses of the drugs in 96% of subjects compared with 16% of controls (P<.001).[67]

Older studies suggest that S chinensis may have a place in the treatment of schizophrenia for amelioration of catatonia, negative symptoms, fatigue, and side effects from neuroleptics and other sedating medications. However, such claims need to be validated by studies using current diagnostic criteria, rigorous methodology, and validated assessment tools before conclusions may be drawn.

Adaptogen Combinations

ADAPT-232 (Chisan), a fixed combination of R rosea, E senticosus, and S chinensis has been used in Scandinavia since 1979 for decreased performance, fatigue, and weakness. Beneficial effects on cognitive functions, attention and memory have been demonstrated in humans using R rosea alone and in combination with other adaptogens.[7] For example, two pilot clinical studies showed that ADAPT-232 significantly improved attention and increased speed and accuracy during stressful cognitive tasks, in comparison to placebo,[16] and significantly decreased the number of mistakes on psychometric tests.[9,57,58]

Preparations and Doses

Preparations and doses of these adaptogens are as follows:

R rosea

Tablets or capsules containing 144 to 200 mg (genuine drug extract ratio [DER] 1.5 to 5:1, extraction solvent ethanol 67% to 70% vol/vol): 144 to 200 mg, daily dose 2 to 4 tablets or capsules. Liquid extract (1:1, ethanol 40% vol/vol): 1 to 3 mL (5–25 drops in a quarter of a glass of water 3 × daily, 15 to 30 minutes before meals). Duration of the treatment: from 10 days to 4 months followed by washout period of 2 weeks.

E senticosus

Total daily dose can be given once a day or in divided doses two or three times daily. Formulations include: tablets or capsules 250 mg; liquid extract (1:1, ethanol 30%–40 % vol/vol) 2–3 mL; dry extracts (ethanol 28%–70% vol/vol) corresponding to 0.5–4 g dried root; dry aqueous extract (15–17:1) 90–180 mg; or tincture: 10–15 mL.

S chinensis

Tablets or capsules (standardized to minimum of 1.3% lignan) 600 to 2000 mg per day; dry extract (DER 1.5 to 5:1, extraction solvent ethanol 67%–70% vol/vol) 144 to 400 mg; and liquid extract (1:1, ethanol 40% vol/vol) 1 to 3 mL (5–25 drops in a quarter of a glass of water 3 times a day, 15–30 minutes before meals).

MECHANISMS OF ACTION AND ACTIVE CONSTITUENTS

Adaptogens increase tolerance to stress and reduce fatigue through effects on mediators of stress response, homeostasis, energy metabolism and the neuroendocrine-immune system. More than 140 compounds have been identified in R rosea roots,[4] 100 in E senticosus roots,[5] and about 200 in S chinensis berries.[6] In vivo and in vitro studies indicate that some isolated constituents (eg, salidrioside, rosavin, tyrosol, eleutheroside E, schizandrin B) contribute to the activity of the whole extracts.[1,9,13–15,30–32]

A recent study demonstrated that the effects of *R rosea, E senticosus, and S chinensis* were associated with upregulation and downregulation of 2188 genes in an isolated human neuroglial cell line T98G. Among these, effects on 260 genes are common to all three plants.[12] Certain isolated constituents affect numerous genes. For example, salidroside (one of the active components of *R rosea*) significantly alters expression of more than 700 genes. Consequently, their pharmacologic activity involves numerous interactions affecting multiple key mediators of stress response and neuroendocrine-immune systems.

Adaptogens are hypothesized to act as "metabolic regulators which increase the ability of an organism to adapt to environmental stressors and prevent damage to the organism by such stressors"[3] at two levels of regulation:

- On the level of whole organism, they support homeostasis and neuroendocrine regulation of the hypothalamic-pituitary-adrenal (HPA) axis (**Fig. 1**),[1,3,10] involving the stress hormones cortisol,[14,25] neuropeptide Y (NPY),[13] and other mediators of stress response, including nitric oxide,[14] membrane bound G-protein receptors,[12] and molecular chaperons heat shock proteins 70 (Hsp70).[11,13]
- On the cellular level, they modulate gene expression (transcriptional control of metabolic regulation) of key mediators of intracellular communications involved in stress-induced signal transduction pathways, including G-protein signaling cyclic adenosine monophosphate (cAMP)-mediated pathway,[12] G-protein signaling phosphatidylinositol, phospholipase C pathways (**Fig. 2**),[12] stress-activated protein kinase JNK (MAPK-9),[11] Hsp70 (stress-protective effect on cellular level),[11,13] heat shock factor 1 (HSF-1),[13] NPY,[13] and Forkhead box O (FOXO) transcription factor[33] (a hypothetical working model for effects of ADAPT-232 on neuroglial cells is available at: http://www.ncbi.nlm.nih.gov/pmc/articles/PMC3269752/pdf/fnins-06-00006.pdf).[13]

See later discussion for the effects of adaptogens on some mediators of stress-response and their functions.

Hsp70: Molecular Chaperones

Hsp70 proteins protect cells from stress-induced damage by temporarily binding to partially-denatured proteins preventing aggregation and allowing their repair and restoration of the three-dimensional structure. Hsp70 participates in disposal of damaged or defective proteins and directly inhibits programmed cell death. ADAPT-232 significantly increased tolerance to stress as demonstrated by the increased endurance of mice in a swim test model.[11] This effect was accompanied by a dramatic increase in serum levels of circulating Hsp70. Similarly, ADAPT-232 and its active constituent, salidroside, stimulated the expression and release of Hsp70 from isolated human neuroglial cells.[13]

NPY

Salidroside and ADAPT-232 stimulate expression and release of NPY from isolated human brain glioblastoma T98G cells,[13] suggesting another important target for adaptogen-mediated stress-protective effects. NPY is a stress-responsive hormone widely distributed in the central and peripheral nervous systems. Sympathoadrenal activation during stress response results in NPY release from sympathetic nerve endings, either alone or with catecholamines. NPY release occurs following stressors such as strenuous exercise and cold exposure, as well as in panic disorder and chronic fatigue syndrome (CFS). The elevation of serum NPY in CFS patients is associated with the severity of stress, negative mood, and clinical symptoms. Furthermore,

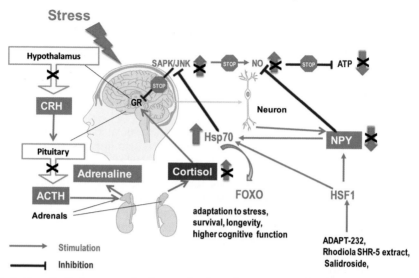

Fig. 1. Hypothetical neuroendocrine mechanism of stress protection by adaptogens (Rhodiola SHR-5 extract, salidroside, ADAPT-232 fixed combination of *R rosea, S chinensis, E senticosus*). Stress induces CRH release from hypothalamus followed by ACTH release from the pituitary, which simulates release of adrenal hormones and NPY to mobilize energy resources and cope with the stress. Feedback regulation of overreaction is initiated by cortisol release from adrenal cortex followed by binding to glucocorticoid receptors (GR) in brain. This signal stops the further release of brain hormones and decreases the stress-induced increase of cortisol down to normal levels. Although short and mild stress (eustress or challenge) is essential to life, severe stress (distress or overload) is associated with extensive generation of oxygen free radicals, including nitric oxide (NO), which is known to inhibit ATP formation (energy-providing molecules). Stress-activated protein kinases (SAPK/JNK/MAPK) inhibit GR, consequently feedback downregulation is blocked and cortisol content in blood remains high in fatigue, depression, impaired memory, ability to concentrate and other stressful conditions. Adaptogens normalize stress-induced elevated levels of cortisol and other extracellular and intracellular mediators of stress response, such as elevated NO, SAPK via upregulation of expression of NPY, heat shock factor (HSF-1) and heat shock proteins Hsp70, which are known to inhibit SAPK. Consequently, NO generation is reduced and ATP production is no longer suppressed. Hsp70 functions intracellularly to enhance antiapoptotic mechanisms, protect proteins against mitochondria-generated oxygen-containing radicals, including nitric oxide and superoxide anion. The released Hsp70 acts as an endogenous danger signal and plays an important role in immune stimulation. Although released NPY plays a crucial role in the HPA axis and maintains energy balance, both NPY and Hsp70 are directly involved in cellular adaptation to stress, increased survival, enhanced longevity and improved cognitive function. Hsp70 inhibits FOXO transcription factor, playing an important role in adaptation to stress and longevity. These pathways contribute to adaptogens effects: antifatigue, increased attention and improved cognitive function. CRH, corticotropin releasing hormone.

psychological stress elevated plasma NPY in healthy subjects. In the periphery, sympathetic nerve-derived and platelet-derived NPY are stimulatory and synergize with glucocorticoids and catecholamines to potentiate the stress response, induce vasoconstriction, and increase vascular smooth muscle cell proliferation. However, in the CNS, NPY acts as an anxiolytic and inhibits sympathetic activity, which results in inhibition of cortisol production by human adrenal cells. NPY can regulate both

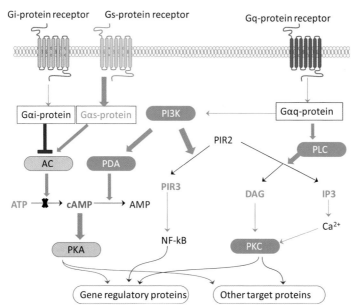

Fig. 2. Hypothetic molecular mechanisms by which adaptogens activate adaptive stress response G-protein coupled receptors (GPCR) pathways. The cell normally receives signals from multiple extracellular stressors that activate cellular signaling pathways (eg, many neurotransmitters activate GPCR). The receptors activate kinase cascades including protein kinases A (PKA), C (PKC), and phosphatidylinositol-3-kinase (PI3K). Adaptogen upregulated proteins are red; downregulated proteins are blue. The gs alpha subunit (Gαs protein) activates the cAMP-dependent pathway by activating adenylate cyclase (AC). The Gi alpha subunit (Gi/G0 or Gi protein) inhibits production of cAMP from ATP. DAG, diacylglycerol; IP3, inositol triphosphate; PLC, phospholipase C. Red arrows indicate activation, blue odd shaped connections indicate inhibition. (*Modified from* Panossian A, Hamm R, Wikman G, et al. Synergy and antagonism of active constituents of ADAPT-232 on transcriptional level of metabolic regulation of isolated neuroglial cells. Front Neurosci 2013, in press.)

immune cells and neuronal cells. For example, NPY strongly inhibits nitric oxide synthesis through Y(1) receptor activation, which prevents interleukin (IL-1β) release and, thus, inhibits nuclear translocation of nuclear factor kappa-light-chain-enhancer of activated B cells (NF-κB), a protein complex that controls transcription of DNA in microglia. NPY plays a protective role in viral infections associated with glial cell activation and production of proinflammatory cytokines in the CNS. It has been suggested that stimulation of NPY gene expression is related to food deprivation and that its overexpression disturbs energy balance leading to increased eating. Within cells, NPY decreases expression of mitochondrial uncoupling protein, thereby promoting adenosyl triphosphate (ATP) formation. NPY stimulates the HPA axis and modulates secretion of hypothalamic neuropeptides.

NPY displayed antidepressant-like activity in the rat forced swimming test. Human studies reveal a role for NPY in "buffering" the harmful effects of stress. Preclinical and clinical evidence suggests mood and cognitive enhancement by NPY. Higher levels of NPY have been observed in soldiers who either present with reduced psychological distress or belong to elite Special Forces. In contrast, decreased levels of NPY were observed in depression and in brain tissues of suicide victims. The antinarcotic effects of adaptogens are mediated by NPY, which plays a role in morphine tolerance and opioid dependence.[13] Morphine significantly decreases NPY levels in the hypothalamus, striatum and adrenal glands. Stress-protective effects of NPY are similar to those of adaptogens.

Pretreatment of human neuroglial cells with NPY-siRNA and HSF1-siRNA significantly suppressed ADAPT-232-induced NPY and Hsp70 release.[13] ADAPT-232-induced expression and release of Hsp70 from glioma cells was dependent on HSF1 or NPY. Thus, HSF1 and NPY may be important upstream molecular targets of adaptogens in neuroglial cells. ADAPT-232 and salidroside act on NPY expression via a mechanism dependent on the upregulation of HSF-1.

ADAPT-232 stimulates secretion of NPY, which influences the HPA axis, energy homeostasis, secretion of Hsp70, cytoprotection, and innate immunity. Hsp70 inhibits FOXO transcription factor, relevant to stress tolerance and longevity. These pathways contribute the antifatigue effect of ADAPT-232, increase attention and improvement in cognitive function. Activation of NPY by ADAPT-232 initiates Hsp70 expression in human neuroglial cells, which maintain homeostasis of neurons. The stimulation and release of stress hormones (NPY and Hsp70) into the blood is an innate defense response to mild stressors (adaptogens), which increases tolerance and adaptation to stress.[13]

Membrane-bound G-protein-coupled Receptors and G-protein-signaling Pathways

The common molecular targets of adaptogens, *R rosea, E senticosus, and S chinensis*, are genes encoding cell membrane bound G-protein-coupled receptors (GPCR), including the 5-HT$_3$ receptor of serotonin and the key proteins of G-protein intracellular signaling downstream pathways: cAMP and phospholipase C/phosphatidylinositol.[12]

GPCRs are involved in many physiologic processes related to stress tolerance, including

- Binding of neurotransmitters involved in regulation of mood, behavior, and cognitive functions, including serotonin, dopamine, GABA, and glutamate
- Regulation of sympathetic and parasympathetic nervous systems responsible for automatic functions, such as blood pressure, heart rate, and digestive processes
- Regulation of immune system activity and inflammation
- Neuroendocrine homeostasis.

Regulation of GPCRs is thought to play a fundamental role in maintaining homeostasis in response to stressors. Many neuropsychiatric drugs either bind directly to specific GPCRs (eg, antipsychotics) or act indirectly via GPCRs by affecting the amount of available agonist (eg, antidepressants). Adaptogens downregulate HTR1A gene encoding the 5-HT3 GPCR that activates an intracellular second messenger cascade to produce excitatory or inhibitory neurotransmission. Serotonin receptors modulate the release of many neurotransmitters, including glutamate, GABA, dopamine, epinephrine, norepinephrine, and acetylcholine, as well as many hormones, including oxytocin, prolactin, vasopressin, cortisol, corticotropin, and substance P. Serotonin receptors influence aggression, anxiety, appetite, cognition, learning, memory, mood, nausea, sleep, and thermoregulation. The binding of serotonin to the 5-HT$_3$ receptor opens membrane channels of neurons in the central and peripheral nervous systems, which in turn leads to an excitatory response and can cause anxiety, a common side effect of serotonin reuptake inhibitors (SSRIs). Downregulation of the HTR1A gene by salidroside and tyrosol (active constituents of *R rosea*) is consistent with the antidepressant effects observed in rat studies,[31,32] and with involvement of serotonin receptors in effects of *R rosea*.[68,69]

Regulation of cAMP and the Activity of Protein Kinase A

Adaptogens reduce the level cAMP and increase the levels of ATP in brain cells possibly by inhibition of adenylate cyclase (synthesis of cAMP) and stimulation of phosphodiesterase (degradation of cAMP). The regulation of the level of cAMP and the activity of protein kinase A (PKA) are key mechanisms for modulation of energy homeostasis and metabolism—the shifting between catabolic and anabolic states. Downregulation of cAMP and PKA by adaptogens decreases stress-induced catabolic transformations and is associated with the stress protective activity of adaptogens. This effect is favorable to ATP-consuming anabolic transformations and provides the rationale for the definition of adaptogens as metabolic regulators.[3] Inhibition of adenylate cyclase by adaptogens can increase intracellular levels of ATP[74] when less of it is converted to cAMP. This may also provide energy for other ATP-dependent enzymatic reactions required for crucial metabolic activities and may contribute to the ability of adaptogens to maintain energy supplies during stress over longer periods of time.

The cells of the prefrontal cortex contain hyperpolarization-activated channels that can open when exposed to cAMP during stress. The excessive opening of these channels impairs higher cognitive function. It has been suggested that inhibitors of cAMP can close the channels, thereby enabling neurotransmission of information connecting neural networks and, thus, improving working memory, which plays a key role in abstract thinking, planning, organizing, and so forth. This mechanism could contribute to the treatment of age-related cognitive decline as well as cognitive disorders in schizophrenia, bipolar disorder, and attention deficit hyperactivity disorder.[34] Such action is consistent with studies showing beneficial effect of ADAPT-232 and Rhodiola on cognitive functions in humans.[7,16,20,24,25,27] For instance, two pilot clinical studies showed that ADAPT-232 significantly improved attention and increased speed and accuracy during stressful cognitive tasks, in comparison to placebo.[16] ADAPT-232 significantly decreased the number of mistakes in complicated psychometric tests[9] and improved the quality-of-life and recovery period of patients suffering from acute nonspecific pneumonia.[24] That is in line also with recent clinical study in which the efficacy of Eleutherococcus in patients with bipolar disorder has been demonstrated.[27]

G-protein-signaling Phosphatidylinositol and Pholpholipase C Pathways

Adaptogens upregulate PLCB1 gene encoding phosphoinositide-specific phospholipase C (PLC) and phosphatidylinositol 3-kinases (PI3Ks) (see **Fig. 2**). G proteins activate phospholipase C (PLC), which catalyzes the hydrolysis of phosphatidylinositol 4,5-bisphosphate (PIP2) into diacyl glycerol (DAG) and inositol-1,4,5-triphosphate (IP$_3$). IP$_3$ is involved in cellular-signaling pathways associated with depression.[70] PI3K is required for long-term potentiation (long-lasting enhancement in signal transmission between neurons), which is critical for memory and learning.[71]

Serpin Peptidase Inhibitor (Neuroserpin)

One more target of adaptogens is the gene SERPIN1 encoding serpin peptidase inhibitor (neuroserpin), which is involved in the development and function of the nervous system and in psychiatric disorders.[72] Neuroserpin plays an important role in the growth of axons, the development of synapses, and the regulation of synaptic plasticity, with implications for learning and memory.[73]

R rosea: Proposed Mechanism of Action in Depression

Although current treatments for depression focus on modulation of monoamines (serotonin and noradrenalin), recent data suggest that antidepressant and stress-protective effects of *R rosea* are related to key mediators of stress response, signal transduction pathways, and regulation of homeostasis. Tyrosol, salidroside (rhodioloside), and rosavin, three of the active constituents in *R rosea*,[11,32] were inactive in (monoamine oxidize) MAOA bioassay. Although another constituent, rosiridin, was found to be the most active inhibitor of MAOA in *R rosea*,[30] it is nearly absent in *R rosea* (SHR-5) extract. Therefore, it is unlikely that the antidepressant activity of *R rosea* is due to MAOA inhibition.

Based on pharmacologic and genomic studies, testable theoretical models for the mechanisms of the antidepressant activity of *R rosea*, salidroside and tyrosol are being developed. Current mechanisms of interest involve effects on

- GPCRs, including 5-HT3 receptor of serotonin
- G protein activated phospholipase C PLC/phosphatidylinositol 4,5-bisphosphate (PIP2) diacyl glycerol (DAG), and IP_3 cellular signaling pathways
- NPY-Hsp70–mediated effects on glucocorticoid receptors, including expression and release of NPY and stress-activated proteins (Hsp70 and JNK).

Proposed mechanisms for effects on cognitive functions, memory, learning, and attention are associated with:

- Downregulation of cAMP followed by closure of hyperpolarization-activated channels
- Activation of PI3K required for long-term potentiation (learning and memory)
- Normalization of cortisol homeostasis
- Genomic effects in neuroglial cells mainly affecting energy metabolism (anabolic effect) and CNS functions, which can be associated with beneficial effects on behavioral, mental and aging related disorders.[12]

SUMMARY

Adaptogenic plants that have been traditionally employed in many countries for centuries require clinical evaluation of their efficacy and safety. In this context, recent clinical trials provide important information for their use in mental and behavioral diseases. Modern research on molecular mechanisms of action is contributing to our understanding of many positive effects of adaptogens, a group of ancient medicinal plants with the potential to improve many aspects of neuropsychiatric disorders, including energy, cognitive function, memory, attention, and mental and physical performance, particularly under stress.

ACKNOWLEDGMENTS

The author acknowledges Dr Gerbarg for her assistance in the preparation of this paper.

APPENDIX: REFERENCES

Supplemental References 35–75 are available at http://www.psych.theclinics.com/dx.doi.org/10.1016/j.psc.2012.12.005.

KEY REFERENCES

1. Panossian A, Wagner H. A review of their history, biological activity, and clinical benefits. HerbalGram 2011;90:52–63.

2. EMEA/HMPC/102655/2007. Reflection paper on the adaptogenic concept. London: European Medicines Agency; 2008.

3. Panossian A, Wikman G, Wagner H. Plant adaptogens III: earlier and more recent aspects and concepts on their modes of action. Phytomedicine 1999;6:287–300.

4. Panossian A, Wikman G, Sarris J. Rosenroot (*Rhodiola rosea*): traditional use, chemical composition, pharmacology, and clinical efficacy. Phytomedicine 2010;17:481–93.

5. Huang L, Zhao H, Huang B, et al. Acanthopanax senticosus: review of botany, chemistry and pharmacology. Pharmazie 2011;66(2):83–97.

6. Panossian A, Wikman G. Pharmacology of *Schisandra chinensis* Bail: an overview of Russian research and uses in medicine. J Ethnopharmacol 2008;118: 183–212.

7. Panossian A, Wikman G. Effects of adaptogens on the central nervous system and the molecular mechanisms associated with their stress—protective activity. Pharmaceuticals 2010;3(1):188–224. Available at: www.mdpi.com/1424-8247/3/1/188/pdf. Accessed October 30, 2010.

8. Panossian A, Wikman G. Evidence-based efficacy of adaptogens in fatigue, and molecular mechanisms related to their stress-protective activity. Curr Clin Pharmacol 2009;4(3):198–219.

9. Panossian A, Wagner H. Stimulating effect of adaptogens: an overview with particular reference to their efficacy following single dose administration. Phytother Res 2005;19:819–38.

10. Panossian A. Adaptogens: tonic herbs for fatigue and stress. Alt Comp Therap 2003;9:327–32.

11. Panossian A, Wikman G, Kaur P, et al. Adaptogens exert a stress-protective effect by modulation of expression of molecular chaperones. Phytomedicine 2009;16: 617–22.

12. Panossian A, Hamm R, Wikman G, et al. Synergy and antagonism of active ingredients of complex herbal preparation ADAPT-232 on transcriptional level of metabolic regulation in isolated neuroglia cells. Front Neurosci 2013.

13. Panossian A, Wikman G, Kaur P, et al. Adaptogens stimulate neuropeptide Y and Hsp72 expression and release in neuroglia cells. Front Neurosci 2012;6:6. http://dx.doi.org/10.3389/fnins.2012.00006. Available at: http://www.frontiersin.org/neuroendocrine_science/10.3389/fnins.2012.00006/full.

14. Panossian A, Hambartsumyan M, Hovanissian A, et al. The adaptogens Rhodiola and Schizandra modify the response to immobilization stress in rabbits by suppressing the increase of phosphorylated stress-activated protein kinase, nitric oxide and cortisol. Drug Target Insights 2007;1:39–54. Available at: www.la-press.com/the-adaptogens-rhodiola-and-schizandra-modifythe-response-to-immobili-a260. Accessed October 16, 2012.

15. Saratikov AS, Krasnov EA. *Rhodiola rosea* (Golden root). 4th edition. Tomsk (USSR): Tomsk State University Publishing House; 2004.

16. Aslanyan G, Amroyan E, Gabrielyan E, et al. Double-blind, placebo-controlled, randomised study of the single dose effects of ADAPT-232 on cognitive functions. Phytomedicine 2010;17:494–9.

17. Darbinyan V, Aslanyan G, Amroyan E, et al. Clinical trial of *Rhodiola rosea* L. extract SHR-5 in the treatment of mild to moderate depression. Nord J Psychiatry 2007;61:2343–8.

18. Dwyer AV, Whitten DL, Hawrelak JA. Herbal medicines, other than St. John's Wort, in the treatment of depression: a systematic review. Altern Med Rev 2011;16(1): 40–9.

19. Edwards D, Heufelder A, Zimmermann A. Therapeutic effects and safety of Rhodiola rosea extract WS® 1375 in subjects with life-stress symptoms—results of an open-label study. Phytother Res 2012;26(8):1220–5.

20. Hartz AJ, Bentler S, Noyes R, et al. Randomized controlled trial of Siberian ginseng for chronic fatigue. Psychol Med 2004;34(1):51–61.

21. Hung SK, Perry R, Ernst E. The effectiveness and efficacy of Rhodiola rosea L.: a systematic review of randomized clinical trials. Phytomedicine 2011;18(4): 235–44.

22. Iovieno N, Dalton ED, Fava M, et al. Second-tier natural antidepressants: review and critique. J Affect Disord 2011;130(3):343–57.

23. Ishaque S, Shamseer L, Bukutu C, et al. Rhodiola rosea for physical and mental fatigue: a systematic review. BMC Complement Altern Med 2012;12:70. http://dx.doi.org/10.1186/1472-6882-12-70.

24. Narimanian M, Badalyan M, Panosyan V, et al. Impact of Chisan® (ADAPT-232) on the quality-of-life and its efficacy as an adjuvant in the treatment of acute non-specific pneumonia. Phytomedicine 2005;12:723–72.

25. Olsson EM, von Schéele B, Panossian AG. A randomized double-blind placebo controlled parallell group study of SHR-5 extract of Rhodiola rosea roots as treatment for patients with stress related fatigue. Planta Med 2009;75:105–12.

26. Spasov AA, Wikman GK, Mandrikov VB, et al. A double-blind, placebo-controlled pilot study of the stimulating and adaptogenic effect of Rhodiola rosea SHR-5 extract on the fatigue of students caused by stress during an examination period with a repeated low-dose regimen. Phytomedicine 2000;7:85–9 [in Russian].

27. Weng S, Tang J, Wang G, et al. Comparison of the addition of Siberian Ginseng (Acanthopanax senticosus) versus fluoxetine to lithium for the treatment of bipolar disorder in adolescents: a randomized. Curt Ther Res Clin Exp 2007;68:280–90.

28. Darbinyan V, Kteyan A, Panossian A, et al. Rhodiola rosea in stress induced fatigue—a double blind cross-over study of a standardized extract SHR-5 with a repeated low-dose regimen on the mental performance of healthy physicians during night duty. Phytomedicine 2000;7:365–71.

29. Shevtsov VA, Zholus BI, Shervarly VI, et al. A randomized trial of two different doses of a SHR-5 Rhodiola rosea extract versus placebo and control of capacity for mental work. Phytomedicine 2003;10:95–105.

30. van Diermen D, Marston A, Bravo J, et al. Monoamine oxidase inhibition by Rhodiola rosea L. roots. J Ethnopharmacol 2009;122:397–401.

31. Panossian A, Nikoyan N, Ohanyan N, et al. Comparative study of Rhodiola preparations on behavioral despair of rats. Phytomedicine 2008;15:84–91.

32. Wikman G, Panossian A. Medicinal herbal extract Carpediol for treating depression. US Patent 6,905,706 B2, June 14, 2005. Filled Apr.16, 2002, p. 1–23.

33. Wiegant FA, Surinova S, Ytsma E, et al. Plant adaptogens increase lifespan and stress resistance in C. elegans. Biogerontology 2009;10:27–42.

34. Wang M, Gamo NJ, Yang Y, et al. Neuronal basis of age-related working memory decline. Nature 2011;476(7359):210–3. http://dx.doi.org/10.1038/nature10243.

St. John's Wort for the Treatment of Psychiatric Disorders

Jerome Sarris, MHSc, PhD[a,b],*

KEYWORDS

- St. John's wort • *Hypericum perforatum* • Herbal medicine • Antidepressant
- Depression • Anxiety • Psychopharmacology • Pharmacogenetics

KEY POINTS

- Evidence supports the use of St. John's wort (SJW) for the treatment of mild-to-moderate depression and somatization disorder, with tentative support in seasonal affective disorder (SAD).
- Evidence does not support the use of SJW for anxiety disorders, attention-deficit hyperactivity disorder (ADHD), or other psychiatric illnesses.
- Differences in the quality and safety of SJW extracts need to be addressed in recommending products to patients.
- Clinicians should be mindful of potential drug interactions if using products with higher (>1 mg) hyperforin and for coadministration with other psychotropic medications.

OVERVIEW

The flowering tops of *Hypericum perforatum* (St. John's wort; SJW) have been used throughout millennia for a range of nervous system conditions, including depressed mood.[1] Dozens of clinical trials have consistently demonstrated the herbal medicine's efficacy in major depressive disorder (MDD). After two randomized controlled trials (RCTs) a decade ago revealed no greater efficacy than placebo,[2,3] clinician enthusiasm for SJW diminished. However, the findings of those studies were not due to a lack of antidepressant efficacy but, instead, reflect a pattern of increasing placebo

---

Disclosure Statement: No direct conflicts noted.

Dr Jerome Sarris is funded by an Australian National Health & Medical Research Council fellowship (NHMRC funding ID 628875), in a strategic partnership with The University of Melbourne and the Center for Human Psychopharmacology at Swinburne University of Technology.

[a] Department of Psychiatry, The Melbourne Clinic, The University of Melbourne, 2 Salisbury Street, Richmond, Victoria 3121, Australia; [b] Centre for Human Psychopharmacology, Swinburne University of Technology, Burwood Road, Hawthorn, Victoria 3122, Australia
* Department of Psychiatry, The Melbourne Clinic, The University of Melbourne, 2 Salisbury Street, Richmond, Victoria 3121, Australia.
E-mail address: jsarris@unimelb.edu.au

Psychiatr Clin N Am 36 (2013) 65–72
http://dx.doi.org/10.1016/j.psc.2013.01.004
0193-953X/13/$ – see front matter © 2013 Elsevier Inc. All rights reserved.

response and decreasing effect sizes, which also exists with conventional antidepressant studies for mild-to-moderate depression.[4,5] This phenomenon may be due to inappropriate recruitment, poor patient selection, inclusion of people with nonbiological depression, or ineligible participants motivated by financial incentives. Although an abundance of SJW MDD studies have been conducted and reviewed in other papers, there is less salient discussion on its clinical applications in other psychiatric disorders. This article outlines the current evidence of the efficacy of SJW in common psychiatric disorders, mechanisms of action, emerging pharmacogenetic data, and clinical and safety considerations.

CLINICAL EVIDENCE
SJW for Depressive Disorders

During the past two decades, more than 40 clinical trials of varying methodological quality have been conducted assessing the efficacy of SJW in treating depressed mood.

Meta-analyses
A meta-analysis of RCTs involving SJW for depression conducted by Linde and colleagues[6] revealed a relative risk (RR) of 1.48 (1.23, 1.77) from 18 combined studies for response to SJW versus placebo and an equivocal effect to selective serotonin reuptake inhibitors (SSRIs) of 1.00 (0.90, 1.15).

A meta-analysis conducted by Rahimi and colleagues[7] found a significant RR for response of 1.22 (1.03, 1.45) in favor of SJW over placebo, with a small weighted mean difference between treatments of 1.33 points (1.15, 1.51) on the Hamilton Depression Rating Scale (HAMD).

Comparison with SSRIs yielded a nonsignificant difference between treatments of 0.32 (−1.28, 0.64) for mean reduction of HAMD score from baseline.

Long-term studies
After 12 weeks of initial treatment in a double-blind RCT by Gastpar and colleagues,[8] subjects continued treatment for up to 24 weeks with either SJW (612 mg per day) or sertraline (50 mg per day). Results revealed that at week 12 both interventions were statistically equivalent; however, at week 24, in the follow-up phase, the mean HAMD score was 5.7 for SJW and 7.1 for sertraline. At the conclusion of the study, 84% of SJW and 81% of sertraline subjects were regarded as responders. It should, however, be noted that sertraline was prescribed at the lower end of the therapeutic range and a greater effect may have occurred at a higher dosage.

A longer term RCT by Kasper and colleagues[9] involving 426 responders (HAMD reduction of 50% or greater) to 6 weeks of SJW (WS 5570) found that, after continuation up to 26 weeks of SJW (900 mg per day) or matching placebo, SJW completers had a relapse rate of 18% (51/282) compared with 25.7% (37 of 144) for placebo. The mean relapse time for SJW was 14 days longer than placebo.

Not all studies are supportive of SJW for the treatment of MDD. The much publicized 2002 National Institute of Mental Health (NIMH)–funded "Hypericum Depression Trial Study Group"[2] (a 3-arm RCT; n = 340) revealed that, at the week 8 endpoint, on the primary outcome measure, neither SJW nor sertraline were significantly different from placebo in reducing HAMD scores. The HAMD total score reduction from baseline to week 8 was −8.68 for SJW versus −10.53 for sertraline and −9.20 for placebo, with no significant difference between groups. A recent analysis showed that, at conclusion of the follow-up part of the trial at week 26, HAMD scores for completers were: sertraline, 7.1; SJW, 6.6; and placebo, 5.7; with no significant difference between treatments.[10]

In other depressive disorders, such as dysthymia and seasonal affective disorder (SAD), clear evidence of efficacy is lacking. A 6-week, 3-arm, RCT of 150 participants with mild-moderate depression (diagnosed using the *Diagnostic and Statistical Manual of Mental Disorders*) was conducted. The subjects took 270 mg of standardized SJW extract PM235 three times a day. Although significant improvement occurred in the nondysthymic subjects, no statistical improvement was revealed in a subanalysis of diagnosed dysthymic subjects on several outcome measures. In respect to SAD, the evidence is only tentatively supportive. Two open-label trials using SJW alone versus light therapy[11] and SJW plus high lux light therapy or low lux control[12] found there was significant reduction of winter-provoked depression for all groups, although there was no statistical difference between the active treatments. Although SJW may be effective in managing SAD, an RCT with an appropriate control is needed for confirmation.

For use in antepartum, peripartum, or postpartum depression, the efficacy of SJW is unclear (see later discussion). Currently, there is no RCT assessing its use in women for this application, and no monotherapy RCT has been conducted examining its use in depression occurring during menopausal transition. There is no firm evidence supporting the efficacy and safety of SJW in treating juveniles with MDD. There are two small ($n = 26$; $n = 33$), 8-week, open-label trials of SJW in juveniles 6 to 17 years old.[13,14] The results of these trials revealed respectable response rates for SJW; however, neither study had a placebo group and there was a high percentage of drop-outs due to continuing depression or noncompliance.

Although it is a commonly held belief that SJW should not be used to treat severe depression, a 6-week RCT involving 251 participants comparing SJW extract WS 5570 (900 mg per day) versus paroxetine (20 mg per day) and placebo in moderate-to-severe depression (HAMD ≥ 22), demonstrated SJW's therapeutic noninferiority (and statistical superiority).[15] The SJW group was found to have a 14.4 decrease on the HAMD compared with an 11.4 decrease for paroxetine. Although this isolated study does support its potential use in nonsuicidal, medication-intolerant patients with more severe depression, SJW is still not advised as a first-line intervention in cases of serious mental illness, or where significant suicidal ideation is present.

SJW for Other Psychiatric Disorders

Aside from application in depression, SJW has been studied in social phobia, obsessive-compulsive disorder (OCD), somatoform disorders, and attention-deficit hyperactivity disorder (ADHD). An open-label study[16] indicated SJW was a promising intervention for use in OCD; however, a more recent controlled study did not support this finding. The RCT recruited 60 participants with a primary diagnosis of OCD to 12 weeks of randomized treatment of SJW (flexible dosing of LI 160; 600 mg–1800 mg depending on response) or matching placebo.[17] Results revealed that the mean reduction on the Yale-Brown Obsessive Compulsive Scale (Y-BOCS) in the active group did not significantly differ from the placebo group. Significant differences were not found on any of the Y-BOCS subscales. In social phobia, one pilot RCT testing SJW (flexible-dose 600–1800 mg daily) in participants with social phobia (assessed via the Liebowitz Social Anxiety Scale) and no comorbid MDD, found no significant differential benefit compared with placebo.[18]

Two RCTs treating somatoform disorders have been conducted. A 6-week multi-center RCT involving 151 subjects with diagnosed somatization or somatoform disorder, found that SJW LI 160 extract (600 mg per day) was significantly superior to placebo in reducing somatoform symptoms demonstrated with a relative −5.17 reduction compared with placebo on the HAMA somatic-subscale item.[19] A 6-week

RCT tested LI 160 SJW extract in 184 subjects with somatization disorders. The results (using six outcome measures) revealed a moderate to large effect size in favor of SJW over placebo on improving somatic symptoms, with 45.4% of the SJW group being classified as responders, compared with 20.9% who took placebo.[20] Improvement in somatic symptoms from SJW correlated with results on the tilt table test. An 8-week RCT has investigated 900 mg daily of standardized SJW or matched placebo in the treatment of 54 children and adolescents with ADHD.[21] Results revealed no significant difference between SJW and placebo on the ADHD Rating Scale-IV, or any attention or hyperactivity subscale **Table 1**.

MECHANISMS OF ACTION OF SJW

SJW contains a range of constituents, including the naphthodianthrones hypericin and pseudohypericin; the phloroglucinol hyperforin; and a range of flavonoids (in free or

Table 1
SJW for the treatment of psychiatric disorders

Psychiatric Condition	Current Evidence	Efficacy	Comment
ADHD	One RCT	X	One negative study; unlikely to be effective
Dysthymia	One RCT	X	One negative study; unlikely to be effective as dysthymia is difficult to treat
Bipolar Disorder	None	?	No studies have been conducted; caution in bipolar disorder unless on mood stabilizers
GAD	None	?	Although anecdotally SJW is commonly used for anxiety, no evidence supports this use
Major Depression	Dozens of RCTs; Meta-analyses	✓	Many positive rigorous RCTs and meta-analyses support the use of standardized high-quality products for MDD
OCD	One open-label study and one RCT	X	Open-label study was positive; however, a high-quality RCT showed no efficacy with SJW
PTSD	None	?	No studies have been conducted; although unlikely to be effective in PTSD
SAD	Two open-label studies	✓	Open-label studies were positive; however, no RCT has been conducted to date
Schizophrenia	None	?	No RCT has been conducted to date; SJW is unlikely to be effective in this condition
Social Phobia	One RCT	X	A high-quality RCT showed no efficacy with SJW
Somatization Disorder	Two RCTs	✓	RCTs were positive, supporting SJW in the treatment of somatization

Abbreviations: ADHD, attention-deficit hyperactivity disorder; GAD, generalized anxiety disorder; OCD, obsessive compulsive disorder; PTSD, posttraumatic stress disorder; SAD, seasonal affective disorder.

glycosidic form), volatile oils, and tannins.[22] Preclinical studies suggest that a range of neurochemical activity is involved with the antidepressant effect of SJW. In vitro and in vivo research has revealed nonselective inhibition of the neuronal re-uptake of serotonin, dopamine, and noradrenalin, and weak monoamine oxidase A and B inhibition.[23] Other biologic activities include a decreased degradation of neurochemicals and a sensitization of and/or increased binding of ligands to various receptors (eg, γ-aminobutyric acid [GABA], glutamate, and adenosine), increased dopaminergic activity in the prefrontal cortex, and neuroendocrine modulation.[1] However, as Cott[24] eruditely comments, the neurochemical effects revealed in preclinical studies have used exceedingly high doses of SJW or its isolated constituents (far above normal clinical doses). Further, the poor bioavailability of many constituents and the lack of penetration across the blood brain barrier (eg, hypericin) suggest that caution needs to be applied when extrapolating from preclinical studies to human clinical activity. One potential mechanism of antidepressant action of SJW could be due to an increased release of monoamines from synaptosomes, thereby affecting neurotransmission via ion channel modulation.[24]

Pharmacogenetic studies are revealing the epigenetic effects of SJW. A recent study evaluated the differential effects of a standardized SJW (0.2% hypericin, 2% hyperforin, 13.3% flavonoids) and fluoxetine on genes involved in the pathogenesis of depression, using a chronic restraint stress model in rats.[25] Analysis of hypothalamic and hippocampal tissue genes found that genes involved with inflammatory processes and oxidative stress were upregulated by both SJW and fluoxetine. A proteomic animal model study conducted by Pennington and colleagues[26] compared the protein expression from SJW to the antidepressant clomipramine and a traditional Chinese medicine formulation, "Xiao-yao-san." From the 1616 protein spots analyzed, SJW was found to differentially express 64 proteins in HT22 cells derived from mouse or rat hippocampal cells, with the most affected involving energy metabolism and axonal outgrowth and regeneration. Wong and colleagues[27] conducted gene expression tests in an animal model comparing 8 weeks of a single daily intravenous dose of imipramine, SJW, or saline control. Results showed that the herb differentially regulated 66 genes and expression sequence tags, whereas imipramine regulated 74 genes. Six common transcripts (concerning synaptic and energy metabolism functions) were expressed by both treatments. An interesting cross-sectional investigation was conducted of the serum brain-derived neurotrophic factor (BDNF) levels in 962 depressed subjects, 700 fully remitted persons (>6 months), and 382 healthy controls.[28] Results revealed that SJW use was significantly associated with higher serum BDNF in depressed patients compared with other medications (although sample size was small).

CLINICAL CONSIDERATIONS IN USE OF SJW

An overarching issue concerning clinicians prescribing any natural medicine is the marked difference in preparation quality and standardization among products.[29] In the case of SJW, results of high quality European pharmaceutical grade extracts cannot be generalized to inferior extracts. Therefore, clinicians are advised to use standardized SJW products, proved effective in clinical trials, to better ensure replication of results. Well-defined SJW products that have been studied include LI-160 (Lichtwer), Ze 117 (Zeller), and WS-5570 (Schwabe). Some of these may be purchased online; however, physician prescription is still advised. The common daily dosage of concentrated SJW is 900 mg, often given in divided doses two to three times per day in tablet form, amounting to about 1.0 mcg of hypericin (the active component) and/or 0.5% to 5% of hyperforin (depending on whether the extract is standardized to reduce hyperforin). However, more severely depressed patients may need up to 1800 mg/day. SJW has not been studied in treatment resistant-depression and it is unlikely in many cases to exert a sufficient thymoleptic effect.

Herb-drug Interactions

Although concerns exist about interactions between SJW and pharmaceuticals, this issue centers on extracts containing higher amounts of hyperforin, which is responsible for inducing cytochrome (CYP) P450 pathways and the P-glycoprotein drug efflux pump; thereby reducing drug serum levels.[30] To illustrate this, a systematic review of 19 studies revealed that high-dose hyperforin extracts (greater than 10 mg per day) had outcomes consistent with CYP3A induction, whereas studies using low-dose hyperforin extracts (less than 4 mg per day) demonstrated no significant effect on CYP3A (thereby lessening the chance of increased metabolism of many common drugs).[31] For this reason, clinicians are advised to only prescribe low hyperforin SJW products if the patient is taking other medication. Products standardized for higher levels of hypericin and flavonoids should not induce CYP pathways.

Risks and Precautions

SJW has a sound safety profile, based on a review of 16 postmarketing surveillance studies ($n = 34{,}834$) that found it to be 10-fold safer than synthetic antidepressants. Furthermore, a meta-analysis noted a significant difference in favor of SJW over conventional antidepressants for discontinuation due to adverse events, with an RR of 0.53 (95% CI: 0.35, 0.82).[7] Aside from rare idiosyncratic reactions, most adverse effects involve reversible dermatologic and gastrointestinal symptoms. Nevertheless, several case reports have reported possible SJW-induced mania, psychosis, and serotonin syndrome.[1] Although many of these mania cases detail concomitant use of other medications and/or recreational drugs, and a background of cyclothymia, a clear temporal association seemed to exist between SJW use and induction of hypomania or mania. Therefore, caution is advised in people with a personal or family history of bipolar disorder. Several case reports of serotonin syndrome have been documented by drug surveillance agencies and this is likely due to use of high dose SJW and/or concomitant use with synthetic antidepressants. Considering this risk, SJW should not be coprescribed with antidepressants. There may be a role for low-dose SJW when a patient is withdrawing from an antidepressant, with the dose being titrated up further when the antidepressant is withdrawn. This needs to occur with appropriate clinical judgment and supervision.

Pregnancy and Lactation

The safe use of SJW during pregnancy and lactation has not been established. An analysis of breast milk from a postpartum lactating mother who was depressed and taking standardized SJW (Jarsin) three times a day, found that only hyperforin was excreted into breast milk, at a very low level.[32] Hyperforin and hypericin were found to be under the lower limit of quantification in the infant's plasma. A prospective study was conducted of 54 SJW exposed pregnancies compared with a matched group of pregnant women taking other pharmacologic therapy for depression and a third matched group of healthy women who were not exposed to any known teratogens.[33] Follow-up information revealed that the rates of major malformations were similar across the three groups, with 5%, 4%, and 0% in the SJW, conventional pharmacotherapy, and healthy groups, respectively ($P = .26$), This was not different from the 3% to 5% risk expected in the general population. However, larger population-based studies would be needed with longer term follow-up evaluation of potential developmental effects to better quantify the risks.

SUMMARY

Current evidence supports the use of high-grade, standardized SJW extracts for the treatment of mild-to-moderate depression and somatization disorder, with tentative support in SAD. Its use cannot currently be extended for anxiety disorders, ADHD, or other psychiatric illnesses. Clinicians should be mindful of potential drug interactions if using products with higher (greater than 1 mg) hyperforin, and in coadministration with other psychotropic medications. SJW should not be prescribed at higher than recommended doses and caution is advised for SJW use in persons with bipolar disorder who are not receiving a mood stabilizer. Future research should explore the use of SJW in generalized anxiety and, potentially, in bipolar depression (adjunctively in patients taking mood stabilizers).

REFERENCES

1. Sarris J, Kavanagh DJ. Kava and St John's wort: current evidence for use in mood and anxiety disorders. J Altern Complement Med 2009;15(8):827–36.
2. Hypericum Depression Trial Study Group. Effect of *Hypericum perforatum* (St John's wort) in major depressive disorder: a randomized controlled trial. JAMA 2002;287(14):1807–14.
3. Shelton RC, Keller MB, Gelenberg A, et al. Effectiveness of St John's wort in major depression: a randomized controlled trial. JAMA 2001;285(15):1978–86.
4. Fournier J, DeRubeis R, Hollon S, et al. Antidepressant drug effects and depression severity: a patient-level meta-analysis. JAMA 2010;303(1):47–53.
5. Werneke U, Horn O, Taylor D. How effective is St John's wort? The evidence revisited. J Clin Psychiatry 2004;65(5):611–7.
6. Linde K, Berner M, Kriston L. St John's wort for major depression. Cochrane Database Syst Rev 2008;(4):CD000448.
7. Rahimi R, Nikfar S, Abdollahi M. Efficacy and tolerability of *Hypericum perforatum* in major depressive disorder in comparison with selective serotonin reuptake inhibitors: a meta-analysis. Prog Neuropsychopharmacol Biol Psychiatry 2009; 33(1):118–27.
8. Gastpar M, Singer A, Zeller K. Efficacy and tolerability of hypericum extract STW3 in long-term treatment with a once-daily dosage in comparison with sertraline. Pharmacopsychiatry 2005;38(2):78–86.
9. Kasper S, Volz HP, Moller HJ, et al. Continuation and long-term maintenance treatment with *Hypericum* extract WS 5570 after recovery from an acute episode of moderate depression—a double-blind, randomized, placebo controlled long-term trial. Eur Neuropsychopharmacol 2008;18(11):803–13.
10. Sarris J, Fava M, Schweitzer I, et al. St John's wort (*Hypericum perforatum*) versus sertraline and placebo in major depressive disorder: continuation data from a 26 week RCT. Pharmacopsychiatry 2012;45(7):275–8.
11. Wheatley D. Hypericum in seasonal affective disorder (SAD). Curr Med Res Opin 1999;15(1):33–7.
12. Martinez B, Kasper S, Ruhrmann S, et al. Hypericum in the treatment of seasonal affective disorders. J Geriatr Psychiatry Neurol 1994;7(Suppl 1):S29–33.
13. Findling RL, McNamara NK, O'Riordan MA, et al. An open-label pilot study of St. John's wort in juvenile depression. J Am Acad Child Adolesc Psychiatry 2003; 42(8):908–14.

14. Simeon J, Nixon MK, Milin R, et al. Open-label pilot study of St. John's wort in adolescent depression. J Child Adolesc Psychopharmacol 2005;15(2):293–301.
15. Szegedi A, Kohnen R, Dienel A, et al. Acute treatment of moderate to severe depression with hypericum extract WS 5570 (St John's wort): randomised controlled double blind non-inferiority trial versus paroxetine. BMJ 2005;330(7490):503.
16. Taylor LH, Kobak KA. An open-label trial of St. John's Wort (Hypericum perforatum) in obsessive-compulsive disorder. J Clin Psychiatry 2000;61(8):575–8.
17. Kobak KA, Taylor LV, Bystritsky A, et al. St John's wort versus placebo in obsessive-compulsive disorder: results from a double-blind study. Int Clin Psychopharmacol 2005;20(6):299–304.
18. Kobak KA, Taylor LV, Warner G, et al. St. John's wort versus placebo in social phobia: results from a placebo-controlled pilot study. J Clin Psychopharmacol 2005;25(1):51–8.
19. Volz HP, Murck H, Kasper S, et al. St John's wort extract (LI 160) in somatoform disorders: results of a placebo-controlled trial. Psychopharmacology (Berl) 2002; 164(3):294–300.
20. Muller T, Mannel M, Murck H, et al. Treatment of somatoform disorders with St. John's wort: a randomized, double-blind and placebo-controlled trial. Psychosom Med 2004;66(4):538–47.
21. Weber W, Vander Stoep A, McCarty RL, et al. Hypericum perforatum (St John's Wort) for attention-deficit/hyperactivity disorder in children and adolescents: a randomized controlled trial. JAMA 2008;299(22):2633–41.
22. Butterweck V, Schmidt M. St. John's wort: role of active compounds for its mechanism of action and efficacy. Wien Med Wochenschr 2007;157(13–14):356–61.
23. Butterweck V. Mechanism of action of St John's wort in depression: what is known? CNS Drugs 2003;17(8):539–62.
24. Cott J. St John's wort. 2nd edition. Informacare; 2010.
25. Jungke P, Ostrow G, Li JL, et al. Profiling of hypothalamic and hippocampal gene expression in chronically stressed rats treated with St. John's wort extract (STW 3-VI) and fluoxetine. Psychopharmacology (Berl) 2010;213(4):757–72.
26. Pennington K, Focking M, McManus CA, et al. A proteomic investigation of similarities between conventional and herbal antidepressant treatments. J Psychopharmacol 2009;23(5):520–30.
27. Wong ML, O'Kirwan F, Hannestad JP, et al. St John's wort and imipramine-induced gene expression profiles identify cellular functions relevant to antidepressant action and novel pharmacogenetic candidates for the phenotype of antidepressant treatment response. Mol Psychiatry 2004;9(3):237–51.
28. Molendijk ML, Bus BA, Spinhoven P, et al. Serum levels of brain-derived neurotrophic factor in major depressive disorder: state-trait issues, clinical features and pharmacological treatment. Mol Psychiatry 2011;16(11):1088–95.
29. Sarris J. Current challenges in appraising complementary medicine evidence. Med J Aust 2012;196(5):310–1.
30. Izzo AA. Drug interactions with St. John's Wort (Hypericum perforatum): a review of the clinical evidence. Int J Clin Pharmacol Ther 2004;42(3):139–48.
31. Whitten D, Myers D, Hawrelak J, et al. The effect of St John's wort extracts on CYP3A: a systematic review of prospective clinical trials. Br J Clin Pharmacol 2006;62(5):512–26.
32. Klier CM, Schafer MR, Schmid-Siegel B, et al. John's wort (Hypericum perforatum)–is it safe during breastfeeding? Pharmacopsychiatry 2002;35(1):29–30.
33. Moretti ME, Maxson A, Hanna F, et al. Evaluating the safety of St. John's Wort in human pregnancy. Reprod Toxicol 2009;28(1):96–9.

Ginkgo biloba
Indications, Mechanisms, and Safety

Bruce J. Diamond, PhD*, Mary R. Bailey, MA

KEYWORDS

- *Ginkgo biloba* • EGb 761 • Antioxidants • Cognitive impairment • Dementia
- Alzheimer disease (AD) • Anti–platelet-activating factor

KEY POINTS

- *Ginkgo biloba* is a medicinal herb used for its purported cognitive and memory-enhancing effects.
- Most randomized control trials use *Ginkgo biloba* special extract EGb761.
- Common clinical indications include Alzheimer and age-associated dementia, cerebral insufficiency, intermittent claudication, and multi-infarct dementia.
- Dosages range from 80 to 720 mg/d with durations ranging from 2 weeks to 2 years.
- Case reports of bleeding are associated with concurrent use of antiplatelet or anticoagulant drugs.
- Potential interactions with monoamine oxidase inhibitors, alprazolam, haloperidol, warfarin, and nifedipine have been reported in case studies.
- Mechanisms of action include increasing cerebral blood flow, antioxidant effects, and antiinflammatory effects.
- Antiplatelet effects have been attributed to flavone and terpene lactone components.
- Although gingko is generally safe, patients should be cautioned regarding possible increased risks of bleeding, particularly when gingko is used with medications exerting synergistic effects.

INTRODUCTION

Ginkgo biloba is one of the most frequently prescribed herbal preparations in Germany and an over-the-counter herbal preparation in the United States.[1] Indications for its use are generally in one of 3 categories: cerebrovascular, peripheral vascular, or tissue damage.[2] Most randomized control trials (RCTs) use the *Ginkgo biloba* special extract EGb 761. Therefore, in this article, the term ginkgo refers to EGb 761, unless otherwise noted.

Disclosure: The authors have no conflicts of interest to disclose.
Neuropsychology, Cognitive Neuroscience, and Clinical Outcomes Laboratory, Department of Psychology, William Paterson University, 300 Pompton Road, Wayne, NJ 07470, USA
* Corresponding author.
E-mail address: diamondb@wpunj.edu

Psychiatr Clin N Am 36 (2013) 73–83
http://dx.doi.org/10.1016/j.psc.2012.12.006
0193-953X/13/$ – see front matter © 2013 Elsevier Inc. All rights reserved.

psych.theclinics.com

COMPOSITION

EGb 761 is standardized to 24% ginkgo-flavone glycosides and 6% terpenoids with the following major constituents (greater than 0.1%): flavonol monoglycosides (eg, quercetin-3-0-glucoside, quercetin-3-0-rhamnoside, and 3'-0-methylmyricetin-3-0-glucoside), flavonol diglycosides, flavonol triglycosides, coumaric esters of flavonol diglycosides, flavonoidic compound, terpenes (eg, bilobalide, ginkgolide A, ginkgolide B, ginkgolide C, ginkgolide J), organic acids, and steroids.

CLINICAL INDICATIONS
Symptoms

Ginkgo's putative neuroprotective and cognitive enhancing properties have provided support for its use in treating neurologic, psychiatric, functional, and physiologic symptoms including problems with memory, information processing, attention and concentration, psychomotor function, mood, fatigue, and activities of daily living.[1,2] Meta-analyses indicate that the cognitive domains yielding the largest proportion of significant effects versus placebo are[3]:

- Fluid intelligence (37.8%)
- Selective attention (43.7%)
- Short-term and long-term verbal and visual memory (ranging from ~28% to 33%) executive functions (eg, planning 33.2%, working memory 20.7%, flexibility 24.4%, and processing speed 33.0%)

In an RCT of patients with multiple sclerosis, ginkgo ameliorated symptoms of fatigue and improved measures of symptom severity and functional outcome. Individuals in the ginkgo group showed more improvement on 4 or more measures with significantly larger effect sizes.[4] In a 4-week RCT involving patients (n = 107, 18–70 years old) with generalized anxiety disorder (GAD) and adjustment disorder with anxious mood, the ginkgo-treated groups (random assignment to 480 mg/d or 240 mg/d) showed a significant dose-dependent reduction on the Hamilton Rating Scale for Anxiety (HAMA) (2.2 and 6.5 points respectively), versus placebo.[5] Effect sizes for GAD were large in both the 480 mg/d group (Cohen's d 5 1.14) and the 240 mg/d group (Cohen's d 5 0.76).[5]

Disorders

Common indications include Alzheimer and age-associated dementia, normal aging, traumatic brain injury, stroke, multi-infarct dementia, cerebral atherosclerosis, cerebral insufficiency, cerebral edema, inflammation, intermittent claudication, and glutamate toxicity,[1] with some work suggesting benefits in multiple sclerosis.[4] In addition, the German Commission E identifies ginkgo for symptomatic treatment of a cluster of disorders including improvement in pain-free walking, peripheral arterial occlusive disease (ie, intermittent claudication), and vertigo and tinnitus of vascular and involutional origin.[2]

A recent study involving 395 patients aged 50 years or older, with probable or possible Alzheimer disease (AD) with cerebrovascular disease and probable vascular dementia (VAD) with neuropsychiatric features, reported that ginkgo (240 mg/d for 22 weeks) showed significant superiority compared with placebo in both types of dementia on the primary outcome measure (Short Syndrome Test and the Stroke Knowledge Test [SKT] cognitive tests battery) and all secondary outcome variables (eg, cognitive, mood, verbal fluency).[6] Ginkgo was equally beneficial in both AD and VAD.[6]

In a double-blind, randomized placebo-controlled (DBRPC), parallel-group, GuidAge clinical trial, 2854 adults in France, aged 70 years or older who spontaneously reported memory complaints were randomly allocated to either 240 mg (twice daily) of ginkgo or matched placebo.[7] Participants were followed for 5 years with the primary outcome, conversion to probable AD in those who received at least 1 dose per day of study ginkgo or placebo.[7] The long-term use of standardized *Ginkgo biloba* extract in this trial did not reduce the risk of progression to AD compared with placebo.[7]

In a multicenter DBRPC 24-week trial in 410 outpatients aged 50 years or older with mild to moderate dementia (AD or VAD) with associated neuropsychiatric symptoms, the subjects were randomly assigned to either 240 mg/d ginkgo or placebo.[8] Subjects treated with ginkgo (n = 200) improved by 2.2 ± 3.5 points (mean ± standard deviation) on the SKT total score, whereas those receiving placebo (n = 202) changed only slightly, by 0.3 ± 3.7 points.[8] The Neuropsychiatric Inventory (NPI) composite score improved by 4.6 ± 7.1 in the ginkgo-treated group and by 2.1 ± 6.5 in the placebo group.[8] Overall, the ginkgo-treated group showed significant and clinically relevant improvement in cognition, psychopathology, functional measures, and quality-of-life scores.[8]

In a community-based, DBRPC, parallel-group trial, 176 participants with mild to moderate dementia were given ginkgo (120 mg/d) or a placebo for 6 months.[9] On primary outcomes (cognitive functioning and participant-rated and career-rated quality of life), the ginkgo group showed no advantage compared with placebo.[9] It should be noted that 120 mg is a lower dose compared with other clinical trials.

In addition to dementia studies, ginkgo has shown some promise as an add-on therapy for symptoms of schizophrenia. In a meta-analysis of 6 studies, 466 cases on ginkgo and 362 cases on placebo were evaluated using the Scale for the Assessment of Negative Symptoms, and the Scale for the Assessment of Positive Symptoms or the Brief Psychiatric Rating Scale.[10] Using standardized mean difference (SMD) scores between pretrial and posttrial scores (and a pooled standard deviation), ginkgo as an add-on to antipsychotic medication produced statistically significant moderate improvement (SMD = −0.50) in total and negative symptoms of chronic schizophrenia, suggesting a role for ginkgo in ameliorating the symptoms of chronic schizophrenia.[10]

DOSAGE AND DURATION

As a dietary supplement, dosages range from 80 mg to 240 mg of dry extract divided into 2 or 3 daily doses, with an average daily recommended dose of 120 mg. The German Commission E recommends 120 to 240 mg of extract 2 to 3 times daily for cerebral insufficiency.[11] Dosages of ginkgo as high as 720 mg/d have been used in clinical trials for dementia, memory, and circulatory disorders.[12] Significant improvement on 1 or more outcome measures is associated with dosages between 120 and 300 mg/d for durations of 3 to 12 weeks.[12] Treatments lasting 4 to 6 weeks are generally needed before positive effects can be expected when ginkgo is taken for disorders of memory, mood, or physiologic function.[1]

MECHANISMS OF ACTION
Overview

Ginkgo seems to exert its effects through its antioxidant and anti–platelet-activating factor (anti-PAF) activity via flavones and terpene lactones, respectively.[1] Ginkgo induces modulatory effects on cerebrovasculature tone, receptor/transmitter activity, glucose metabolism, and electroencephalographic activity.[1]

Cerebral Blood Flow

The terpene lactones (ginkgolides) inhibit PAF and facilitate blood flow.[12] Pretreatment with high doses of ginkgo may decrease reperfusion injury, improving cardiac index and left ventricular stroke work following aortic valve replacement, although clinical outcomes may not differ.[11] Ginkgo can exert arterial and venous vasoactive changes associated with increases in tissue perfusion, peripheral and cerebral blood flow, ocular blood flow and microcirculation.[2]

Meta-analysis indicates a positive effect of ginkgo on blood perfusion, providing support for its use in peripheral artery occlusive disease as well as tinnitus and vertigo of vascular origin.[13] Vasoregulation, platelet antagonism, and protection against post-ischemic oxidative damage seem to be primary mechanisms mediating ameliorative effects in intermittent claudication.[11]

Metabolism, Antioxidation, and Antiinflammatory Properties

Improving blood flow, reducing ischemia-reperfusion injury, and inhibiting platelets are putative mechanisms in vascular dementia. In AD, hypothesized neuroprotective mechanisms include antioxidation, antiapoptosis, antiinflammation, protection against mitochondrial dysfunction, amyloidogenesis and amyloid β aggregation, ion homeostasis, modulation of phosphorylation of tau protein, and possibly induction of growth factors.[14]

Abnormalities in mitochondrial function are associated with the pathologic changes seen in AD. Ginkgo may have direct protective effects on mitochondria that contribute to its antioxidant effects because the mitochondrial respiratory chain is both the major target and source of reactive oxygen species (ROS). Flavonoids scavenge ROS. However, extrapolating from in vitro and in vivo animal models to clinical applications is difficult and the mechanisms underlying the potential protective effects of ginkgo and its constituents on mitochondrial function need further clarification.

Evidence that ginkgo may protect against mitochondrial dysfunction is based on findings that abnormalities in mitochondrial function are associated with the pathologic changes in AD.[14] Ginkgo may also provide antiapoptotic actions via intracellular signaling pathways involved in apoptosis, with flavonoid and terpene fractions playing a prominent role.[14]

Human Imaging Work

Examination of possible inhibition of monoamine oxidase (MAO) A and B using positron emission tomography imaging after 1 month of treatment with ginkgo 120 mg/d revealed no change in either MAO A or B levels,[2] suggesting that ginkgo did not cross the blood-brain barrier. It was hypothesized that differences between in vitro and in vivo animal and human models may be based on the pharmacology, pharmacokinetics, and pharmacodynamics of ginkgo components, in addition to animal studies using larger dosages than clinical trials (**Table 1**).

MAGNITUDE AND MEANING OF TREATMENT EFFECTS

Determining the clinical significance of treatment effects is complex because of differences in outcome measures, measurement sensitivity, and lack of standardization across studies. Outcomes that are statistically significant may not be clinically significance.[1] In contrast, findings that fail to reach statistical significance (compared with a healthy control group, published norms, or previous baseline performance) may not reflect effects on disease progression (ie, in AD).[1] Overall, clinically meaningful,

Table 1
Summary of *Ginkgo biloba* studies

Reviews/Meta-analyses	Clinical Indications	Methods	Subjects	Dosage and Duration	Mechanisms of Action	Adverse Events	Conclusions
Diamond et al,[1] 2000	MID, DAT Neuroprotective cognitive function Cerebrovascular insufficiency, ischemia Vestibular disorders Tinnitus, hypoxia Intermittent claudication	DBRCTs and SBRCTs	24 studies from n = 8 to n = 309	120–300 mg/d for 3–12 wk (noticeable effects usually begin after 4–6 wk)	Anti-PAF Calcium channels Vasomodulatory ↑ Glucose uptake Antioxidant	Case studies of bleeding Headache Gastrointestinal upset, nausea	Promising DAT, traumatic brain injury, stroke, normal aging, edema, tinnitus, macular degeneration. Caution with anticoagulants
Ponto and Schultz,[2] 2003	VAD, DAT Maintain healthy CNS functioning Enhance cognitive functioning	RCTs, animal studies	9 RCTs from n = 60 to n = 214 3 rat studies	120 mg/d for 4+ wk 240 mg/d for 4+ wk (effects usually 4–6 wk)	Antioxidant ↑ Cerebral blood flow	Gastrointestinal, headache Dermal hypersensitivity Case studies of bleeding	Inconclusive efficacy in enhancing cognition in healthy adults
Valli and Giardina,[11] 2002	Cerebrovascular and peripheral vascular disease, sexual dysfunction, hearing affective disorders Multiple sclerosis Retinal disorders memory and cognition	Case reports	n = 1	120–160 mg/d 120–240 mg/d Duration not cited	Antiplatelet Antioxidant Antiinflammatory Vasodilation ↓ Blood viscosity ↓ Ischemia-reperfusion injury	Nausea, dyspepsia Headache Case studies of hematoma, hemorrhage, or hyphema	May improve intermittent claudication and benefit cerebrovascular disease. Additional research recommended

(continued on next page)

Table 1
(continued)

Reviews/Meta-analyses	Clinical Indications	Methods	Subjects	Dosage and Duration	Mechanisms of Action	Adverse Events	Conclusions
Bressler,[12] 2005	Dementias, Tinnitus, Anxiety, Raynaud disease	DBRCTs	20 studies ranging from n = 99 to n = 415	80–240 mg/d Duration not discussed	Neuroprotective, Antioxidant	Headache, dizziness, Gastrointestinal, Heart palpitations, Allergic reaction, Seeds can be lethal	Ginkgo improving memory is inconclusive, Possible drug interactions
Kellermann and Kloft,[13] 2011	Tinnitus, Peripheral artery disease, Dementias, Cognitive function	RCT	n = 1985	80–240 mg/d, 1 wk to 6 y	Neuroprotective, Antioxidant, Decreased blood viscosity	No general risk of bleeding but case studies cite ↓ blood viscosity	No general risk of bleeding
Bent et al,[16] 2005	Dementia, tinnitus, vertigo, Asthma/allergies, Cerebrovascular disease, Memory	Case report	n = 1	80–600 mg/d, 1 wk to 2 y	Vasodilation, Antioxidant, Inhibits PAF	Case studies of bleeding, headache, Nausea, confusion	Possible interaction ↑ Risk of bleeding, but more support needed
Napryeyenko et al,[6] 2009	VAD, DAT	RCT	n = 395	240 mg/d, 22 wk	Not discussed	Headache, Dizziness, abdominal pain, Nausea, influenza, Angina pectoris, More adverse events on placebo	Cognitive performance significantly improved
Vellas et al,[7] 2012	DAT	DBRCT	n = 2854	240 mg/d, 5 y	Antioxidant	Stroke, Cardiac disorders, Hemorrhagic event	Long-term ginkgo did not inhibit development of DAT

Study	Condition	Study type	n	Dosage	Mechanism	Adverse events	Outcomes
Woelk et al,[5] 2007	Dementias	DBRCT	n = 107	480 mg or 240 mg/d, 4 wk	Not discussed	Gastroenteritis Tachycardia with hypertension	Anxiety significantly reduced by ginkgo
Johnson et al,[4] 2006	Memory deficits Depression Cerebral insufficiency Tinnitus, fatigue Anxiety	DBRCT	n = 22	240 mg/d, 4 wk	Antioxidant Vascular modulation Regulates glucose metabolism and cerebrovascular tone	None reported	Improved fatigue, symptom severity, and functionality
Herrschaft et al,[8] 2012	Dementias	DBRCT	n = 410	240 mg/d, 24 wk	Mitochondrial regulation Neuroprotective	Headache, dizziness Hypertension Abdominal pain Drowsiness	Improved cognition and psychopathology
McCarney et al,[9] 2008	Dementia	DBRCT	n = 176	120 mg/d, 6 mo	Not discussed	Gastrointestinal Cardiac and vascular effects	No general cognitive improvements
Singh et al,[10] 2010	Schizophrenia (ginkgo used as an add-on therapy)	RCTs	6 studies: n = 466 ginkgo n = 362 placebo	From 120 mg/d to 360 mg/d, >8 wk	Antioxidant Inhibits PAF	Gastrointestinal upset, nausea Headache Dizziness Allergic reaction	Efficacy as adjunct in schizophrenia
Kaschel,[3] 2009	Dementia, tinnitus, Cognitive function Vertigo, depression Multiple sclerosis Intermittent claudication	DBRCTs	29 RCTs from n = 24 to n = 240	From 80 mg/d to 240 mg/d, greater than 4 wk	Antioxidant Neuroprotective Inhibits PAF	Adverse events not discussed	Improved selective attention, long-term memory, executive processing

Abbreviations: CNS, central nervous system; DAT, dementia of the Alzheimer type; DBRCT, double-blind RCT; MID, multi-infarct dementia; SBRCT, single-blind RCT; VAD, vascular dementia.

although subtle, improvements have been observed in several studies across causes and indications.[1]

CONCENTRATION-DEPENDENT EFFECTS AND EFFICACY

Flavone, ginkgolide B, bilobalide, and ginkgolide A are the principal components of ginkgo that are thought to exhibit concentration-dependent antioxidant, metabolic, and neurotransmitter, regulatory effects.[1] Many studies support ginkgo's efficacy and safety in healthy and clinical populations.[1] However, no effects, selective effects, and effects that run counter to predicted outcomes have also been reported.[1] Some studies suggest that gingko may be no more effective than either nicergoline or dihydroergotoxine in treating cerebrovascular disease, and several studies have reported that it is not effective in treating vascular dementia and vertigo (See more recent work in section on Disorders).[1]

ADVERSE EVENTS

Most studies reporting side effects have been case reports with dosages ranging from 80 to 150 mg/d for durations of 1 week to up to 1 year, with many patients having comorbid conditions and taking other medications. Several case studies report bleeding abnormalities that are potentially attributable to ginkgo,[2] including reports suggesting that ginkgo may cause postoperative bleeding.[15] The mechanism of action may involve the constituents ginkgolide, bilobalide, and other components that are PAF receptor antagonists.

Analysis of RCTs involving adults with dementia, peripheral artery disease, or diabetes mellitus show positive effects of ginkgo on blood perfusion (by significant reduction in blood viscosity) but no significant effect on adenosine 5′-diphosphate–induced platelet aggregation, fibrinogen concentration, activated partial thromboplastin time, and prothrombin time, suggesting no higher bleeding risks associated with standardized ginkgo extract.[13]

Taken together, the evidence is equivocal for a causal association between ginkgo use and changes in blood coagulation parameters. Most patients had other clinical risk factors and only a small percentage of cases provided information on bleeding times.[10] A conservative treatment approach should be mindful of possible increased risks of bleeding, particularly when ginkgo is used with medications exerting anticoagulant effects.[15]

DRUG INTERACTIONS
Antiplatelet Drugs

Unusual bleeding has been attributed to the inhibition of PAF via the ginkgolide B component, leading to cautions regarding the concomitant use of ginkgo with drugs exhibiting antiplatelet activity (eg, aspirin, nonsteroidal antiinflammatory drugs, and anticoagulants).[2] Ginkgo may interact with warfarin, resulting in an enhancement of warfarin's effects by decreasing clearance and increasing bioavailability.[2] Case reports have described intracerebral hemorrhage following initiation of ginkgo in an individual taking warfarin for several years, and blurred vision and spontaneous bleeding from the iris into the anterior chamber of the eye in another individual taking aspirin (acetylsalicylic acid).[16] Bleeding ended after ginkgo was discontinued.[16] Ginkgolides, which are terpene lactones with anti–platelet-activating activity, may be mediating factors.[16] Some reports suggest that bleeding can occur when ginkgo is taken in combination with drugs that affect platelet function and/or coagulation (eg, ibuprofen or rofecoxib).[11,12,15] Serious adverse events were reported with concurrent use of aspirin (spontaneous hyphema), warfarin (intracerebral hemorrhage), and ibuprofen (comatose state with intracerebral mass bleeding), but recent trials have not confirmed these effects.[15] Systematic reviews of case reports conclude that causal relationships between ginkgo intake and bleeding are unlikely, and a review of RCTs does not show changes in blood coagulation parameters.[15]

Calcium Channel Antagonists

A theoretically based interaction in an animal model has been reported with nicardipine and ginkgo resulting in an attenuation of the hypotensive response of nicardipine via a mechanism involving the induction of CYP3A2 and other liver metabolizing enzymes, although dosage levels were higher than standard human dosages.[17] Although clinical interactions are not substantiated, caution may be warranted with the use of long-term, high-dose ginkgo extract and calcium channel antagonists, which are metabolized by the same enzymes.[17]

Depression

Trazodone, which is used in treating depression in the elderly when sedation is required, has been suspected of interacting with ginkgo in a patient with AD, resulting in a coma.[17] However, this conclusion remains unproven.[17]

Herbs and Surgery

Ginkgo may have the potential to interact with drugs that are used during surgery, but the effect of herbal medicines on the response to anesthetics has not been fully

Table 2 Drug interactions	
Drug	**Adverse Reaction/Interactions**
Warfarin (Coumadin, Jantoven, Marfarin), ibuprofen (Advil), aspirin, vitamin E	Case study: bleeding[11,12,15–17]
Rofecoxib (Vioxx)	Case study: bleeding[15,17]
Antiplatelets and anticoagulants	Case studies: bleeding[15]
Antiepileptics	Seizure in 1 case report[15]
Thiazides	Increased blood pressure in 1 case report[15]
Midazolam (Versed)	Mixed results in 4 pharmacokinetic trials[15]
Omeprazole (Losec, Prilosec, Omesec)	Reduced drug concentration in pharmacokinetic trials[12,15]
Risperidone (Risperdal)	Priapism in 1 case report[15]
Ritonavir (Norvir)	Decreased AUC in 1 pharmacokinetic trial[15]
Tolbutamide (Orinase, Tol-Tab)	Mixed results in 2 pharmacokinetic trials[15]
Trazodone (Desyrel, Oleptro)	Coma in 1 case report[11,15,17] Increased sedative effects[12]
Alprazolam (Xanax, Niravam)	Decreased AUC[12,15]
Nicardipine (Cardene)	Possible interaction at high doses[17]
MAOIs	Synergistic effects[1]
Haloperidol (Haldol)	Increased effectiveness[12]
Nifedipine (Adalat, Afeditab CR, Nifediac)	Increased effectiveness[11]

Abbreviations: AUC, area under the curve; MAOI, monoamine oxidase inhibitor.

evaluated.[17] The American Society of Anesthesiologists has recommended that all herbal medications be stopped 2 to 3 weeks before elective surgery, with ginkgo specifically identified because it may increase bleeding (**Table 2**).[17]

SUMMARY AND FUTURE DIRECTIONS

Future research needs to address the issue that dosages used in many animal studies are often not representative of human dosage ranges and that reactions to ginkgo reflect many factors including pharmacology, pharmacokinetics, and pharmacodynamics of individual ginkgo components in addition to possible synergistic effects.[2] Statements of efficacy are complicated by diverse methodologies, measures, and analysis techniques, arguing for controlled trials with more sensitive and standardized outcome measures, validated inter-rater and intrarater reliability, test-retest reliability, parallel test forms, and more detailed patient descriptions and diagnoses. Future research should quantify and characterize ginkgo bioavailability, washout periods, and long-term effects, and determine the following:

1. Dose-response characteristics
2. Optimal timing and duration for treatment interventions and its use as an adjunctive therapy
3. Conditions and symptoms for which ginkgo is most and least useful
4. Possible drug interactions

Ginkgo has been studied in numerous controlled trials and has displayed a good safety profile over time. It has shown potential in ameliorating the effects of a variety of disorders and symptoms. Mechanisms of action have been examined and expressed in multiple studies using both human and animal models, and possible drug interactions and adverse events continue to be explored in clinical trials.

In summary, ginkgo has the potential to provide a safe alternative and complementary tool in treating a variety of symptoms and disorders. Patient outcomes, safety, and research are optimized when clinicians and researchers are informed with respect to composition, indications, disorders, dosages/durations, mechanisms, concentration-dependent effects and efficacy, adverse events, and possible drug interactions.

REFERENCES

1. Diamond BJ, Shiflett SC, Feiwel N, et al. Ginkgo biloba extract: mechanisms and clinical indications. Arch Phys Med Rehabil 2000;81:668–78.
2. Ponto LL, Schultz SK. Gingko biloba extract: review of CNS effects. Ann Clin Psychiatry 2003;15:109–19.
3. Kaschel R. Ginkgo biloba: specificity of neuropsychological improvement? A selective review in search of differential effects. Hum Psychopharmacol 2009; 24:345–70.
4. Johnson S, Diamond BJ, Rausch S, et al. The effect of gingko biloba on functional measures in multiple sclerosis: a pilot randomized controlled trial. Explore (NY) 2006;2:19–24.
5. Woelk H, Arnoldt K, Kieser M, et al. Ginkgo biloba special extract EGb 761 in generalized anxiety disorder and adjustment disorder with anxious mood: a randomized, double-blind, placebo-controlled trial. J Psychiatr Res 2007;41: 472–80.
6. Napryeyenko O, Sonnik G, Tartakovsky I. Efficacy and tolerability of Ginkgo biloba extract EGb 761 by type of dementia: analyses of a randomised controlled trial. J Neurol Sci 2009;283:224–9.

7. Vellas B, Coley N, Ousset P, et al. Long-term use of standardised ginkgo biloba extract for the prevention of Alzheimer's disease (GuidAge): a randomised placebo-controlled trial. Lancet Neurol 2012;11:851–9.
8. Herrschaft H, Nacu A, Likhachev S, et al. Ginkgo biloba extract EGb 761 in dementia with neuropsychiatric features: a randomised, placebo-controlled trial to confirm the efficacy and safety of a daily dose of 240 mg. J Psychiatr Res 2012;46:716–23.
9. McCarney R, Fisher P, Iliffe S, et al. Ginkgo biloba for mild to moderate dementia in a community setting: a pragmatic, randomised, parallel-group, double-blind, placebo-controlled trial. Int J Geriatr Psychiatry 2008;23:1222–30.
10. Singh V, Singh SP, Chan K. Review and meta-analysis of usage of ginkgo as an adjunct therapy in chronic schizophrenia. Int J Neuropsychopharmacol 2010;13:257–71.
11. Valli G, Giardina EV. Benefits, adverse effects and drug interactions of herbal therapies with cardiovascular effects. J Am Coll Cardiol 2002;39:1083–95.
12. Bressler R. Interactions between ginkgo biloba and prescription medications. Geriatrics 2005;60:30–3.
13. Kellermann AJ, Kloft C. Is there a risk of bleeding associated with standardized ginkgo biloba extract therapy? A systematic review and meta-analysis. Pharmacotherapy 2011;31:490–502.
14. Shi C, Liu J, Wu F, et al. Ginkgo biloba extract in Alzheimer's disease: from action mechanisms to medical practice. Int J Mol Sci 2010;11:107–23.
15. Izzo AA, Ernst E. Interactions between herbal medicines and prescribed drugs: an updated systematic review. Drugs 2009;69:1777–98.
16. Bent S, Goldberg H, Padula A, et al. Spontaneous bleeding associated with ginkgo biloba. J Gen Intern Med 2005;20:657–61.
17. Williamson EM. Drug interactions between herbal and prescription medicines. Drug Saf 2003;26:1075–92.

Saffron, Passionflower, Valerian and Sage for Mental Health

Amirhossein Modabbernia, MD,
Shahin Akhondzadeh, PhD, FBPharmacolS*

KEYWORDS

- *Crocus sativus* • *Passiflora incarnata* • *Salvia officinalis* • *Valeriana officinalis*
- Anxiety • Insomnia • Depression • ADHD

KEY POINTS

- Saffron, traditionally valued as a spice, has been studied as a potential antidepressant and cognitive enhancer.
- Passionflower is widely used for its reputed sedative/anxiolytic properties.
- The efficacy of valerian as a herbal sedative is only weakly supported by research evidence.
- Sage has been reported to improve cognitive function and reduce agitation in patients with mild to moderate Alzheimer disease.

INTRODUCTION

This article discusses the quality of evidence supporting mental health benefits and risks of 4 widely used herbal medicines: saffron (*Crocus sativus*), passionflower (*Passiflora incarnata*), valerian (*Valeriana officinalis*), and sage (*Salvia officinalis*).

SAFFRON (*C SATIVUS*)

Saffron, the world's most expensive spice, is derived from the flower of *C sativus*. Originating in Crete, *C sativus* has been used for thousands of years and is mentioned in a seventh century BC Assyrian botanic text. Although it has been propagated throughout Eurasia and other continents, Iran produces 90% of the world's saffron and generates most of the research into its potential medical uses.[1,2]

Conflicts of Interest: None.
Psychiatric Research Center, Roozbeh Hospital, Tehran University of Medical Sciences, South Kargar Street, Tehran 13337, Iran
* Corresponding author. Psychiatric Research Center, Roozbeh Hospital, South Kargar Street, Tehran 13337, Iran.
E-mail address: s.akhond@neda.net

Depression

There are 5 published randomized controlled trials (RCTs; total n = 190, 6–8 weeks), all of which show the beneficial effects of monotherapy with saffron stigma or petal (30 mg/d in 2 or 3 divided doses) in depression.[3–7] Saffron was as efficacious as imipramine (100 mg/d) and fluoxetine (20 mg/d) and more efficacious (mean reduction on Hamilton Scale of 12–14 points) than placebo in treatment of mild to moderate depression. Saffron was as well tolerated as fluoxetine and better tolerated than imipramine. Reuptake inhibition of monoamines, N-methyl-D-aspartate (NMDA) antagonism, and possibly improved brain-derived neurotrophic factor signaling might be implicated in the antidepressant mechanisms of action of saffron.[8] Taken together, saffron monotherapy is an efficacious and tolerable strategy for treatment of mild to moderate depression with a moderate to high quality of evidence.

Reproductive and Sexual Problems

An RCT of saffron (15 mg twice a day for 2 menstrual cycles) for premenstrual syndrome showed significantly more efficacy than placebo in improving depression and other premenstrual symptoms.[9] In an open-label study (n = 35), saffron aroma reduced cortisol levels and anxiety, and increased estrogen levels in both follicular and luteal phases.[10] Administration of saffron stigma to 20 patients with erectile dysfunction for 10 days at high dose (200 mg/d) significantly improved nocturnal penile tumescence and sexual function scores.[11] In an RCT of 30 depressed men with fluoxetine-induced sexual dysfunction, saffron (15 mg twice a day) significantly improved erectile function and intercourse satisfaction, but not desire or orgasmic function.[12] Also, in an RCT of 34 women with fluoxetine-associated sexual dysfunction, saffron stigma improved arousal, pain, and lubrication domains, but not satisfaction, orgasm, or desire.[13]

Alzheimer Disease

Evidence suggests that saffron both antagonizes glutamatergic activity on NMDA receptors (as does memantine)[8] and inhibits acetylcholinesterase (as does donepezil).[14] Moreover, saffron has shown neuroprotective and anti-inflammatory properties.[15] In a 16-week RCT of 46 patients with mild to moderate Alzheimer disease (AD), saffron 15 mg twice a day was associated with significantly more improvement in cognitive function than placebo. Tolerability of saffron was similar to that of placebo.[16] In a 22-week RCT, saffron 15 mg twice daily was as efficacious as donepezil 5 mg twice daily, but caused fewer side effects.[16]

Adverse Effects and Toxicity

In a 1-week RCT on healthy volunteers (n = 30), high doses of saffron (400 mg/d but not 200 mg/d) reduced systolic blood pressure (10 mm Hg) and mean arterial pressures (5 mm Hg) significantly. It also induced slight but clinically insignificant changes in blood and biochemical parameters.[17] However, with usual clinical doses (less than 100 mg/d), saffron is as tolerable as placebo.[18] In light of 1 reported case of anaphylaxis, saffron should be ruled out as a possible allergen when taking a history in cases of allergic reactions.[19]

PASSIONFLOWER (P INCARNATA)

Passionflower is a woody, hairy, climbing vine that has been included in herbal remedies, mainly as a liquid tincture.[1] It has traditionally been used as a mild anxiolytic and sedative hypnotic.

Anxiety

In an RCT comparing the effect of *P incarnata* 45 drops/d and oxazepam 30 mg/d in 36 patients with generalized anxiety disorder (GAD), both drugs were equally effective in reducing anxiety. *P incarnata* showed a delayed onset of action (day 7) compared with oxazepam (day 4), whereas more impairment of job performance was seen with oxazepam.[20] In 2 placebo-controlled RCTs, administration of *P incarnata* 90 minutes before outpatient surgery (500 mg) or 30 minutes before spinal anesthesia (700 mg) reduced anxiety levels without impairing psychomotor function.[21,22]

The *P incarnata* extract modulated both gamma-aminobutyric acid (GABA) A and B receptors without interacting with the ethanol and benzodiazepine sites of the GABA-A receptor.[23]

Sleep

An RCT (n = 41) found that *P incarnata* herbal tea significantly enhanced subjective sleep quality but not polysomnographic measures compared with placebo.[24] Further controlled studies using objective measures of sleep quality are needed to validate this finding.

Symptoms of Substance Withdrawal

A placebo-controlled RCT (n = 65) in patients with opioid addiction found greater improvement in mental symptoms in those who received *P incarnata* (60 drops/d) add-on to clonidine (maximum of 0.8 mg/d) than in those who received a placebo add-on.[25]

Toxicity

P incarnata has been listed as a safe herbal sedative by the US Food and Drug Administration and most drug monographs; however, one drug preparation (Relaxir) containing *P incarnata* was associated with altered consciousness in 5 individuals. It is generally advised not to take *P incarnata* along with central nervous system stimulants or depressants.[26] Because of 1 report of prolonged corrected QT interval and episodes of ventricular tachycardia in a 34-year old woman following self-administration of therapeutic doses of *P incarnata*,[27] caution is suggested in recommending *P incarnata* to patients with cardiac abnormalities.

VALERIAN (*V OFFICINALIS, VALERIANA EDULIS*)

Valerian is a hardy perennial plant, with sweetly scented pink or white flowers that bloom during the summer.[1] Known to Hippocrates and Galen, it has traditionally been used for insomnia, anxiety, seizures, and migraine.

Sleep

Although preliminary evidence had suggested moderate sedative activity for *V officinalis*, the most recent systematic review (18 RCTs including 2 large studies) found little objective evidence for the benefits of valerian in sleep problems, whereas it showed improved subjective sleep quality compared with placebo. Therefore, it was suggested that other more promising treatment strategies should be used before trying valerian for sleep.[28]

Anxiety

A 4-week placebo-controlled RCT compared the effects of placebo (n = 12), *V officinalis* extract (mean dose 81.3 mg/d; n = 12), and diazepam (6.5 mg/d; n = 12) in patients with GAD. Compared with placebo, patients who received valerian or diazepam had significant improvement in HAM-A psychic factor (but not total anxiety scores), suggesting modest benefit in anxiety.[29]

Obsessive-Compulsive Disorder

An 8-week double-blind RCT showed that V officinalis (765 mg/d) in patients with obsessive-compulsive disorder (OCD) significantly improved symptoms compared with placebo. The only frequent side effect in the valerian group was somnolence.[30]

Adverse Effects and Toxicity

A systematic review of 37 studies (including 23 controlled trials) of valerian for insomnia found the herb to be safe but not efficacious.[31] Valerian can potentiate sedative drugs, which can result in an increased risk of falls in the elderly. Valerian inhibited cytochrome P450 enzymes 3A4, 2D6, and 2C19 in vitro, and there are some reports that suggest hepatotoxicity in humans.[32] Therefore, it is advisable to avoid valerian administration to patients with liver disease. In animals, up to 65 times the human dose of V officinalis did not result in adverse reproductive outcomes. Human studies are needed to confirm these findings.[33]

SAGE (S OFFICINALIS)

S officinalis is an evergreen perennial bush, with grayish leaves, woody stems, and blue to purplish flowers. Native to the Mediterranean region, it has naturalized in many places throughout the world.[1]

Dementia

S officinalis inhibits cholinesterase, exerts protective effects against cellular damage, and improves mood and cognition in animals and healthy human subjects.[34] In a 4-month double-blind RCT in patients with mild to moderate AD, S officinalis (60 drops/d) yielded significantly better cognitive performance and less agitation compared with placebo.[35]

Adverse Events and Toxicity

Short-term and medium-term use of sage is generally well tolerated. Like other aromatic plants, sage contains thujone, which can cause severe nervous system symptoms such as convulsions and hallucinations. Severe side effects are uncommon with a daily intake of thujone of less than 0.11 mg/kg/d (2–20 cups of sage tea).[36] Tonic clonic seizure following accidental consumption of sage oil has been reported in children.[37]

SUMMARY

This article reviews the use of saffron, sage, passionflower, and valerian in mental health treatment. Saffron has shown beneficial effects for patients with mild to moderate depression and mild to moderate AD, and is probably beneficial sexual dysfunction and premenstrual syndrome. Studies of the effects of passionflower in the treatment of sleep and anxiety disorders have been promising. It has also been successfully used as a calming agent before surgery and as an adjunct to clonidine in the treatment of substance withdrawal. Valerian offers modest benefit for treatment of anxiety and sleep disorders. Sage improved symptoms of dementia in 1 study, though the study needs replication.

REFERENCES

1. Akhondzadeh S. Herbal medicine in the treatment of psychiatric and neurological disorders. In: L'Abate L, editor. Low cost approaches to promote physical and mental health: theory research and practice. New York: Springer; 2007. p. 119–38.
2. Kamalipour M, Jamshidi AH, Akhondzadeh S. Antidepressant effect of *Crocus sativus*: an evidence based review. Journal of Medicinal Plants 2010;9(Suppl 6): 35–8.
3. Akhondzadeh Basti A, Moshiri E, Noorbala AA, et al. Comparison of petal of *Crocus sativus* L. and fluoxetine in the treatment of depressed outpatients: a pilot double-blind randomized trial. Prog Neuropsychopharmacol Biol Psychiatry 2007;31(2):439–42. http://dx.doi.org/10.1016/j.pnpbp.2006.11.010.
4. Akhondzadeh S, Fallah-Pour H, Afkham K, et al. Comparison of *Crocus sativus* L. and imipramine in the treatment of mild to moderate depression: a pilot double-blind randomized trial [ISRCTN45683816]. BMC Complement Altern Med 2004;4: 12. http://dx.doi.org/10.1186/1472-6882-4-12.
5. Akhondzadeh S, Tahmacebi-Pour N, Noorbala AA, et al. *Crocus sativus* L. in the treatment of mild to moderate depression: a double-blind, randomized and placebo-controlled trial. Phytother Res 2005;19(2):148–51. http://dx.doi.org/10.1002/ptr.1647.
6. Moshiri E, Basti AA, Noorbala AA, et al. *Crocus sativus* L. (petal) in the treatment of mild-to-moderate depression: a double-blind, randomized and placebo-controlled trial. Phytomedicine 2006;13(9–10):607–11. http://dx.doi.org/10.1016/j.phymed.2006.08.006.
7. Noorbala AA, Akhondzadeh S, Tahmacebi-Pour N, et al. Hydro-alcoholic extract of *Crocus sativus* L. versus fluoxetine in the treatment of mild to moderate depression: a double-blind, randomized pilot trial. J Ethnopharmacol 2005;97(2):281–4. http://dx.doi.org/10.1016/j.jep.2004.11.004.
8. Berger F, Hensel A, Nieber K. Saffron extract and trans-crocetin inhibit glutamatergic synaptic transmission in rat cortical brain slices. Neuroscience 2011;180: 238–47. http://dx.doi.org/10.1016/j.neuroscience.2011.02.037.
9. Agha-Hosseini M, Kashani L, Aleyaseen A, et al. *Crocus sativus* L. (saffron) in the treatment of premenstrual syndrome: a double-blind, randomised and placebo-controlled trial. BJOG 2008;115(4):515–9. http://dx.doi.org/10.1111/j.1471-0528.2007.01652.x.
10. Fukui H, Toyoshima K, Komaki R. Psychological and neuroendocrinological effects of odor of saffron (*Crocus sativus*). Phytomedicine 2011;18(8–9): 726–30. http://dx.doi.org/10.1016/j.phymed.2010.11.013.
11. Shamsa A, Hosseinzadeh H, Molaei M, et al. Evaluation of *Crocus sativus* L. (saffron) on male erectile dysfunction: a pilot study. Phytomedicine 2009;16(8): 690–3. http://dx.doi.org/10.1016/j.phymed.2009.03.008.
12. Modabbernia A, Sohrabi H, Nasehi AA, et al. Effect of saffron on fluoxetine-induced sexual impairment in men: randomized double-blind placebo-controlled trial. Psychopharmacology (Berl) 2012. http://dx.doi.org/10.1007/s00213-012-2729-6.
13. Kashani L, Raisi F, Saroukhani S, et al. Saffron for treatment of fluoxetine-induced sexual dysfunction in women: randomized double-blind placebo-controlled study. Hum Psychopharmacol 2012, in press. http://dx.doi.org/10.1002/hup.2282.
14. Geromichalos GD, Lamari FN, Papandreou MA, et al. Saffron as a source of novel acetylcholinesterase inhibitors: molecular docking and in vitro enzymatic studies. J Agric Food Chem 2012;60(24):6131–8. http://dx.doi.org/10.1021/jf300589c.

15. Nam KN, Park YM, Jung HJ, et al. Anti-inflammatory effects of crocin and crocetin in rat brain microglial cells. Eur J Pharmacol 2010;648(1–3):110–6. http://dx.doi.org/10.1016/j.ejphar.2010.09.003.
16. Akhondzadeh S, Sabet MS, Harirchian MH, et al. Saffron in the treatment of patients with mild to moderate Alzheimer's disease: a 16-week, randomized and placebo-controlled trial. J Clin Pharm Ther 2010;35(5):581–8. http://dx.doi.org/10.1111/j.1365-2710.2009.01133.x.
17. Modaghegh MH, Shahabian M, Esmaeili HA, et al. Safety evaluation of saffron (Crocus sativus) tablets in healthy volunteers. Phytomedicine 2008;15(12):1032–7. http://dx.doi.org/10.1016/j.phymed.2008.06.003.
18. Mansoori P, Akhondzadeh S, Raisi F, et al. A randomized, double-blind, placebo-controlled study of safety of the adjunctive saffron on sexual dysfunction induced by a selective serotonin reuptake inhibitor. Journal of Medicinal Plants 2011;10(37):121–30.
19. Wuthrich B, Schmid-Grendelmeyer P, Lundberg M. Anaphylaxis to saffron. Allergy 1997;52(4):476–7.
20. Akhondzadeh S, Naghavi HR, Vazirian M, et al. Passionflower in the treatment of generalized anxiety: a pilot double-blind randomized controlled trial with oxazepam. J Clin Pharm Ther 2001;26(5):363–7.
21. Aslanargun P, Cuvas O, Dikmen B, et al. Passiflora incarnata Linneaus as an anxiolytic before spinal anesthesia. J Anesth 2012;26(1):39–44. http://dx.doi.org/10.1007/s00540-011-1265-6.
22. Movafegh A, Alizadeh R, Hajimohamadi F, et al. Preoperative oral Passiflora incarnata reduces anxiety in ambulatory surgery patients: a double-blind, placebo-controlled study. Anesth Analg 2008;106(6):1728–32. http://dx.doi.org/10.1213/ane.0b013e318172c3f9.
23. Appel K, Rose T, Fiebich B, et al. Modulation of the gamma-aminobutyric acid (GABA) system by Passiflora incarnata L. Phytother Res 2011;25(6):838–43. http://dx.doi.org/10.1002/ptr.3352.
24. Ngan A, Conduit R. A double-blind, placebo-controlled investigation of the effects of Passiflora incarnata (passionflower) herbal tea on subjective sleep quality. Phytother Res 2011;25(8):1153–9. http://dx.doi.org/10.1002/ptr.3400.
25. Akhondzadeh S, Kashani L, Mobaseri M, et al. Passionflower in the treatment of opiates withdrawal: a double-blind randomized controlled trial. J Clin Pharm Ther 2001;26(5):369–73.
26. Dhawan K, Dhawan S, Sharma A. Passiflora: a review update. J Ethnopharmacol 2004;94(1):1–23. http://dx.doi.org/10.1016/j.jep.2004.02.023 pii: S0378874104000856.
27. Fisher AA, Purcell P, Le Couteur DG. Toxicity of Passiflora incarnata L. J Toxicol Clin Toxicol 2000;38(1):63–6.
28. Fernandez-San-Martin MI, Masa-Font R, Palacios-Soler L, et al. Effectiveness of valerian on insomnia: a meta-analysis of randomized placebo-controlled trials. Sleep Med 2010;11(6):505–11. http://dx.doi.org/10.1016/j.sleep.2009.12.009 pii: S1389-9457(10)00100-0.
29. Andreatini R, Sartori VA, Seabra ML, et al. Effect of valepotriates (valerian extract) in generalized anxiety disorder: a randomized placebo-controlled pilot study. Phytother Res 2002;16(7):650–4. http://dx.doi.org/10.1002/ptr.1027.
30. Pakseresht S, Boostani H, Sayyah M. Extract of valerian root (Valeriana officinalis L.) vs. placebo in treatment of obsessive-compulsive disorder: a randomized double-blind study. J Complement Integr Med 2011;8(1). http://dx.doi.org/10.2202/1553-3840.1465.

31. Taibi DM, Landis CA, Petry H, et al. A systematic review of valerian as a sleep aid: safe but not effective. Sleep Med Rev 2007;11(3):209–30. http://dx.doi.org/10.1016/j.smrv.2007.03.002.
32. Vassiliadis T, Anagnostis P, Patsiaoura K, et al. Valeriana hepatotoxicity. Sleep Med 2009;10(8):935. http://dx.doi.org/10.1016/j.sleep.2008.09.009 pii: S1389-9457(08)00276-1.
33. Yao M, Ritchie HE, Brown-Woodman PD. A developmental toxicity-screening test of valerian. J Ethnopharmacol 2007;113(2):204–9. http://dx.doi.org/10.1016/j.jep.2007.05.028.
34. Akhondzadeh S, Abbasi SH. Herbal medicine in the treatment of Alzheimer's disease. Am J Alzheimers Dis Other Demen 2006;21(2):113–8.
35. Akhondzadeh S, Noroozian M, Mohammadi M, et al. *Salvia officinalis* extract in the treatment of patients with mild to moderate Alzheimer's disease: a double blind, randomized and placebo-controlled trial. J Clin Pharm Ther 2003;28(1): 53–9.
36. Lachenmeier DW, Uebelacker M. Risk assessment of thujone in foods and medicines containing sage and wormwood–evidence for a need of regulatory changes? Regul Toxicol Pharmacol 2010;58(3):437–43. http://dx.doi.org/10.1016/j.yrtph.2010.08.012 pii: S0273-2300(10)00139-X.
37. Halicioglu O, Astarcioglu G, Yaprak I, et al. Toxicity of *Salvia officinalis* in a newborn and a child: an alarming report. Pediatr Neurol 2011;45(4):259–60. http://dx.doi.org/10.1016/j.pediatrneurol.2011.05.012 pii: S0887-8994(11)00217-7.

Science of the Mind
Ancient Yoga texts and Modern Studies

Shirley Telles, MBBS, PhD (Neurophysiology)*, Nilkamal Singh, MSc

KEYWORDS

- Yoga • Science • Ancient texts • Evidence-based findings

KEY POINTS

- Concepts about yoga in ancient texts can sometimes be verified by research.
- Breathing is an important link between body and mind.
- Yoga breathing techniques and meditation influence physical and mental functions.
- Recent research techniques have revealed interesting mechanisms underlying the effects.
- Yoga voluntarily regulated breathing techniques vary based on their rate and depth, among other factors.

INTRODUCTION

Ancient yoga practices are being studied with modern scientific techniques as we try to understand their effects on physical and emotional states. This article begins with basic yoga concepts and focuses on the effects of rapid yoga breathing and single-nostril breathing on metabolism and neurologic function. Recent brain imaging studies reveal the impact of yoga postures and meditation on brain activity. For a discussion of the neurophysiology and clinical uses of slower breath techniques, see the article *Breathing Practices for Treatment of Psychiatric and Stress-related Medical Conditions* by Brown, Gerbarg, and Muench in this issue. Additional analysis of research on meditation is presented in this issue by Marchand: *Buddhism, Mindfulness, MBSR, MBCBT* and by Fehmi and Shor: *Open Focus*.

Concepts of Yoga and Schools of Yoga Both Ancient and Modern

Yoga is an ancient way of life, which was intended to help individuals consciously evolve spiritually.[1] There are several definitions of yoga, which, when put together, give an idea about this complex practice.

Yoga has been defined as the process of gaining mastery over fluctuations in the mental state (*Yogah chitta vrtti nirodhah*, Patanjali's Yoga Sutras, Chapter 1, Verse

Conflict of Interest: Nil.

Department of Research on Yoga, Patanjali Research Foundation, Haridwar, Uttarakhand 249405, India
* Corresponding author.
E-mail address: shirleytelles@gmail.com

Psychiatr Clin N Am 36 (2013) 93–108
http://dx.doi.org/10.1016/j.psc.2013.01.010
0193-953X/13/$ – see front matter © 2013 Elsevier Inc. All rights reserved.

2; Patanjali circa 900 BC). This Sutra suggests that yoga practice helps to reach a state of calm as mentioned in an earlier text (the *Bhagavad Gita*), which states that yoga is synonymous with equilibrium or balance (*Samatvam yoga uchayate, Bhagavad Gita,* Chapter 2, Verse 48, *Bhagavad Gita* compiled circa 500 BC). However, yoga was never intended to be associated with inactivity. Thus, the same text describes yoga as "skill in action" (*Yogah karmasu kaushalam, Bhagavad Gita,* Chapter 2, Verse 50). From this it is apparent that yoga practitioners can carry out whatever activity they are required to, while certain practices and a particular mental attitude help them to remain calm and in a state of balance or homeostasis.

The sage Patanjali made the first attempt to compile several descriptions of yoga practices and their effects systematically. This compilation suggests that there are 8 limbs,[2] as follows:

1. A moral code of conduct or *yama*
2. Self-purification and study or *niyama*
3. Physical postures or *asanas*
4. Voluntary breath regulation or *pranayamas*
5. Sense withdrawal or *pratyahara*
6. Concentration or *dharana*
7. Meditation or *dhyana*
8. Absorption in the self or *samadhi*

From this compilation, it is interpreted that from physical practices (physical postures and voluntary breath regulation) one gradually progresses toward regulating the mental states (concentration, meditation, absorption in self).

Following sage Patanjali's description of the 8 limbs of yoga intended to help attain *Samadhi* or total freedom, a more recent philosopher and visionary, Swami Vivekananda (1863–1902), expanded the definition of yoga to cover diverse aspects of life.[3] He conceptualized 4 ways of practicing yoga as a part of life that resemble the 8 steps of *ashtanga* described by Patanjali:

1. Performing work with a selfless attitude (*karma yoga*)
2. Getting an in-depth knowledge about life and spirituality (*jnana yoga*)
3. Surrendering to a Supreme force (*bhakti yoga*)
4. Yoga practices for spiritual growth (*raja yoga*)

In the last hundred years numerous yoga schools or ways of teaching have emerged. Some are named after yoga masters, such as Iyenger yoga after B.K.S. Iyenger, and Bikram Yoga, after Bikram Choudhary. The names of other schools are based on the method or practices involved, for example, *Kriya yoga,* popularized by Paramahamsa Yogananda, and *Hatha yoga,* used to describe any method that places an emphasis on physical practices.

This diversity in yoga methods is important because it meets the needs of widely differing yoga aspirants. Many yoga practices can help achieve the same result, such as a calm mental state and spiritual growth.

LINKS BETWEEN MIND AND BODY: CONCEPTS IN YOGA TEXTS AND MODERN SCIENCE
The Importance of Breathing and the Way in Which Breathing Influences the Mind

All life processes require some form of energy; hence, organisms that are able to obtain and use the energy they need efficiently are likely to have a better chance to survive in a competitive environment.[4] The ancient Indian Science of Yoga places a definite emphasis on respiration and respiratory control. In some of the ancient texts

(The *Upanishads*, circa 1500 BC), the way in which a person breathes is considered important for a spiritual aspirant to reach their goal.[5]

Breath regulation is given this importance in yoga because it is believed to influence the mental state and hence the overall functioning. According to one of the *Upanishads,* this has been described more clearly.[6] This description states that there are 5 levels of existence: (1) the physical level, (2) the level of subtle energy (called *prana* in Sanskrit), (3) the instinctual mental level, (4) the intellectual mental level, and (5) a state of optimal health and homeostasis. Imbalances are believed to occur at the mental level when there is conflict between the instinct and the intellect.[1,7] The first obvious sign of this imbalance is at the level of subtle energy, which results in irregular breathing. In *Patanjali's Yoga Sutras* (Chapter 1, Verse 31) it is stated that "the manifestations of a distracted mental state are mental anguish, tremors, rough and erratic breathing and general nervousness." It is believed, but not proven, that if a person realizes at this stage that something is wrong, they may be able to make the necessary physical and mental changes to prevent disease. For this reason, internal and external awareness are such an important part of yoga practice. Hence early detection and correction of erratic breathing could possibly prevent disease. Modern research on the health benefits of breath practices supports this belief, although more studies are needed to identify and validate the specific practices and their impact on disease progression.

Another yoga text (*Hatha Yoga Pradipika*, circa 300 AD) also places importance on the breath as a way to influence the mental state. It is stated, "when the breath (used interchangeably with *prana*) is irregular the mental state is erratic; when the breath is steady the mental state is steady as well. By this practice the yogi attains stability and hence should regulate the breath" (*Hatha Yoga Pradipika*, Chapter 2, Verse 2).

Scientific Evidence Supporting the Link Between Breath Regulation and the Mental State

Prototypical respiratory-facial-postural responses to 6 basic emotions were described from several physiologic reactions present in people reliving intense emotional experiences.[8,9] Respiratory movement and facial/postural expression were recorded from 36 actors who had learned previously to express these emotions with prototypical actions. A qualitative analysis of the recording showed that, as the emotions were reproduced, both breathing and expression evolved from an initial robot-like face to a more natural stage characterized by spontaneous vocalizations and gestures. Quantitatively well-differentiated sets of respiratory changes characterize 6 basic emotions. Conversely, concurrent activation of the respiratory-facial-postural systems can generate the same emotions. Hence, not only are specific emotions characterized by distinct respiratory patterns but breathing in those patterns can generate these emotions.[10]

PHYSIOLOGIC EFFECTS OF VOLUNTARILY REGULATED YOGA BREATHING PRACTICES

Voluntarily regulated yoga breathing techniques (VRYB) are called *pranayamas*. This term derives from Sanskrit, where *prana* means "life energy," "vital energy," or even "breath," and *ayama* means "to prolong." There are several types of *pranayama* practices, which differ in the way they modify breathing, involving the following:

1. Changes in rate
2. Changes in the nostril through which the person breathes
3. Exhalation during which a sound is produced
4. Changes in the volume of air taken in

5. Breathing with a constricted glottis
6. Breathing with a period of breath-holding
7. Breathing through the mouth

The physiologic effects of many voluntarily regulated breathing practices have been studied as well as their influence on different systems within the body.

Effects on Metabolism

Metabolism is most easily quantified or measured by studying oxygen consumption. Early studies[11,12] measured oxygen consumption using a closed circuit apparatus, whereas more recent studies use the less cumbersome and more natural open circuit apparatus.[13] VRYB with breath-holding influences the metabolism in a unique way. When the period of breath-holding (called *kumbhak*, meaning "a pot" in Sanskrit) was shorter than that of inhalation or exhalation (breath rate, 5–7 bpm), oxygen consumption increased by 56%.[11] In contrast, when the period of breath-holding was longer than the period of inhalation or exhalation (breath rate, 1.5–2.5 bpm), oxygen consumption decreased by 19%.

Apart from VRYB with breath-holding, practices involving uninostril (unilateral nostril) breathing and alternate nostril breathing also influence metabolism. For example, the immediate effect of 45 minutes of right uninostril yoga breathing (breath rate, 8–12 bpm) was also an increase in oxygen consumed along with sympathetic activation.[14] Right uninostril yoga breathing practiced for 1 month for 45 minutes each day also increased oxygen consumption and sympathetic activation.[12] On the other hand, alternate nostril yoga breathing (breath rate, 7–9 bpm) reduced metabolic rate, heart rate, and systolic blood pressure when practiced for 4 weeks.[15] More recently, alternate nostril yoga breathing has been shown to reduce systolic and mean blood pressure.[16]

Another VRYB that influences the metabolism is a high-frequency yoga breathing (HFYB) called *kapalabhati*, which literally means "shining forehead" in Sanskrit. This technique involves active exhalation at an increased breath rate. Practicing HFYB for 15 minutes resulted in an increase in energy expenditure. During the practice of HFYB, the major portion of the energy was derived from carbohydrates and, following HFYB, the major source of energy was from fats.[13] These studies showed that various VRYB techniques have different effects on metabolism, which could be mediated by the hypothalamus, endocrine glands, autonomic nervous system, or other mechanisms.

Effects on the Nervous System

Evaluation of the effects of VRYB on the nervous system have been based on performance in attention and memory tasks, spontaneous electrical activity (electroencephalogram), evoked electrical activity (evoked potentials and event-related potentials), and cerebral blood flow as indicated by transcranial Döppler and functional near infrared spectroscopy.

Cancellation tasks are used to measure selective attention, concentration, and visual scanning. Improved performance in the cancellation task was noted following right uninostril breathing and alternate nostril breathing[17] and after 2 minutes of HFYB.[18] Studies on the effects of VRYB on memory have been limited to uninostril yoga breathing to determine whether these practices influence the ipsilateral or contralateral cerebral hemisphere.[19] Using spatial and verbal memory tasks, it was found that right, left, or alternate nostril yoga breathing all led to improvement in spatial memory, which is a right-hemisphere–specific task, suggesting that, irrespective of the nostril, uninostril yoga breathing causes changes in the right cerebral hemisphere.[20] Sympathetic activation, which is required for vigilance, may contribute to effects on attention and memory.[21] Several studies on VRYB have shown an increase in sympathetic nervous system activity based on heart rate variability as well as skin conductance and cutaneous blood flow. HFYB practiced at 120 bpm and right uninostril breathing increased sympathetic nervous system activity.[14,22] In contrast, HFYB at 60 bpm, alternate nostril breathing, and breathing out with a humming sound (*Bhramari pranayama;* breath rate, 10–12 bpm) showed either an absence of sympathetic activation[23] or a decreased sympathetic activity with increased parasympathetic activity.[22,24] Breathing out while chanting the Sanskrit syllable OM (breath rate, 10–12 bpm) was associated with decreased heart and breath rates and increased skin conductance.[25]

Electroencephalogram studies of central nervous system activity during VRYB, particularly during *bhramari pranamaya*, found paroxysmal gamma waves,[26] a pattern that has been correlated with meditative mental states.

Evoked potential studies have allowed approximate spatial localization of neural correlates of breathing practices. Auditory evoked potentials were recorded during VRYB with partial closure of the glottis creating airway resistance (*ujjayi pranayama*, which means "victorious breath" in Sanskrit; breath rate, 7–9 bpm).[27] This VRYB was followed by better transmission of auditory information at the level of the thalamus. A similar result was seen following breathing out with the sound OM.[28] Right uninostril breathing showed evoked potential changes localized to the right cerebral hemisphere and right subcortical regions.[29] The P300 event-related potential has been administered before and after specific VRYB as a measure of attention task performance. Following HFYB there was a significant improvement in the P300 auditory oddball task performance[30] and better performance in a letter cancellation task.[18] Following right, left, and alternate nostril yoga breathing, the P300 potential was improved from a site recorded over the right hemisphere compared with the left hemisphere. Hence, similar to auditory evoked potentials, this auditory event-related potential task showed an ipsilateral change with right uninostril breathing.[31]

These changes in evoked potentials and event-related potentials suggest that specific brain areas are activated with particular VRYB. Normally, changes in the functions of specific brain areas are associated with either global or localized changes in cerebral blood flow depending on the area of activation.[32] Cerebral blood flow following HFYB was assessed in 2 separate studies using transcranial Döppler and functional near-infrared spectroscopy. Both studies showed no change in cerebral blood flow, which is to be expected as the cerebral blood flow is well regulated.[33] However, the functional near-infrared spectroscopy study did show increased deoxy-hemoglobin over the dorsolateral prefrontal cortex with decreased oxyhemoglobin, suggesting that this part of the brain showed focal activation.[34] This study is consistent with results suggesting that HFYB facilitates performance in an attention task because the dorsolateral prefrontal cortex is involved in executive functions, including attention.[35]

Effects of VRYB on Perception and Motor Performance

The previous section described effects of VRYB on the functioning of the nervous system. Hence it is not surprising that these practices can enhance sensory perception, contributing to greater sensitivity to stimuli as well as a wider interpretation of a sensory stimulus.[36,37] HFYB improved visual and tactile perception immediately after 15 minutes of practice.[36] Also, following HFYB, visual perception improved with a decrease in the degree of perceived optical illusion. It is unclear whether the change was at the level of the sensory organ (the eye) or primary relay centers such as the thalamus, and/or whether it was due to cognitive-judgmental factors.[37] Reflex responses to sensory stimuli improved following 3 minutes of a rapid forceful type of breathing called bellows breath (*bhastrika pranayama*; breath rate, 5–7 bpm).[38] Elementary school boys who practiced bellows-type breathing showed a significant decrease in both visual and auditory reaction time. Following alternate nostril yoga breathing, patients with hypertension showed improvement in another kind of performance, finger dexterity.[39]

Mechanism of Action for Voluntarily Regulated Yoga Breathing Techniques

VRYB with breath-holding lowered chemosensitivity to hypercapnia,[40] suggesting an effect on the neural control of breathing. VRYB techniques without breath-holding improved the functioning of the respiratory muscles and had several beneficial effects on lung capacity and on the small airways.[41] Apart from these physical effects, VRYB can change mental states. Numerous mechanisms are being studied to generate testable hypotheses that may explain how VRYB affects acute mental states, emotion regulation, cognitive function, recovery from psychological stressors, and long-term character development. For example, voluntary slow breathing stretches the lung tissue, producing inhibitory signals from 2 sources,[42] slowly adapting receptors and hyperpolarizing currents. These inhibitory signals are believed to activate neurons simultaneously within the hypothalamus, leading to changes in the autonomic nervous system with increased parasympathetic dominance and reduced metabolism. Other VRYB practices that involved right uninostril breathing caused sympathetic arousal. This sympathetic arousal is believed to be mediated in part via the hypothalamus. Several of the effects of VRYB are probably due to the interaction between the respiratory centers in the brain stem and the hypothalamus. In panic disorder, dysregulation of both the respiratory control systems and the hypothalamic pituitary adrenal axis have been implicated. Individuals with panic disorder were found to have elevated levels of adrenocorticotropic hormone and persistent irregularities in tidal volume because of the frequent occurrence of sighs.[43] Regression analysis showed that tidal volume irregularities and the frequency of sighs were strongly predicted by levels of adrenocorticotropic hormone before any challenge. Most VRYB techniques regularize or pace breathing.[2] Because there is a report of reduced levels of cortisol following Sudarshan Kriya yoga breathing (a present day derivation of *bhastrika pranayama*),[44] it could be one of the ways in which physiologic stress reduction occurs. It is also essential to emphasize that the VRYB techniques should be practiced correctly, which is mentioned in one of the ancient yoga texts (ie, *Hatha Yoga Pradipika*, Chapter 2, Verse 16, "By the proper practice of *pranayama* all diseases are eradicated while through the improper practice of *pranayama* all diseases can occur").[45] Details about the method of practice for VRYB, the precautions, and contraindications are provided in **Table 1** and the applications are provided in **Table 2**.

YOGA-BASED MEDITATION AND MIND BODY REGULATION
Physiologic Effects Emphasizing the Nervous System

The early studies of transcendental meditation reported a shift toward parasympathetic dominance with a wakeful but relaxed mental state.[46] To a large extent, this description seems to be validated in current studies of several meditation techniques. However, studies of some meditation techniques find increases in sympathetic activity.[47–49] It has been hypothesized that these inconsistent findings could be because in some studies practitioners were in a state of focused attention (FA), whereas in other studies practitioners were in a state of open monitor meditation (OM).[50] Although the FA state is presumably associated with sympathetic activation, the OM state may be associated with parasympathetic activity. Interestingly, Patanjali (circa 900 BC) described states corresponding to FA and OM. The *dharana* state means "confining the mind within a limited mental area" (*Desha bandhash cittasya dharana*, Patanjali's Yoga Sutras, Chapter 3, Verse 1) and is more comparable to the FA state. The next stage of meditation described by Patanjali is *dhyana*, which is an "uninterrupted flow of the mind toward the object chosen for meditation" (*Tatra Pratyayaikatanata dhyanam*, Patanjali's Yoga Sutras, Chapter 3, Verse 2). This state conforms reasonably well to the description of an OM state. Recent studies have shown that the physiologic effects of meditative focusing (*dharana*) and meditation (*dhyana*) are different from one other. The practice of *dhyana* was associated with signs of reduced sympathetic nervous system activity based on heart rate variability, skin conductance, and cutaneous blood flow.[51] Also, in meditation (*dhyana*) auditory evoked potentials showed no changes at the level of the brain stem.[52] Furthermore, the speed of sensory transmission was reduced in the thalamus and cortex.[53] The main effect of meditative focusing (*dharana*) was to improve the performance in a letter cancellation task, which requires attention.[54] Hence descriptions of meditative states in ancient texts of either the Buddhist or the yoga traditions can provide clues to guide research on the physiologic effects of meditation.

Recent techniques have been used to assess both the immediate and the long-term effects of yoga practice. Gamma amino butyric acid (GABA)-to-creatinine ratios were measured using magnetic resonance spectroscopic imaging immediately before and immediately after a 60-minute yoga *asana* session (n = 8) and a 60-minute reading session (n = 11).[55] There was a 27% increase in levels of GABA in the yoga practitioner group after the yoga session but no change in the comparison group. In a subsequent study by the same authors, yoga *asana* practitioners (n = 19) were compared with a group who practiced metabolically matched walking (n = 15).[56] The yoga group reported greater improvement in mood and a greater decrease in anxiety along with an increase in levels of thalamic GABA. These 2 reports examined practitioners of yoga postures or *asanas* using magnetic resonance spectroscopy. Magnetic resonance imaging has been used to assess long-term anatomic changes in meditation practitioners.[57] There were 16 meditation-naïve participants and 17 in a wait-list control group. Both groups were assessed using anatomic magnetic resonance images. After an 8-week program of mindfulness-based stress reduction, the meditators showed an increase in the gray matter concentration in the left hippocampus (as a priority region of study), whereas whole brain analysis showed an increase in the posterior cingulate cortex, the temporo-parietal junction, and the cerebellum, in the meditators compared with the controls. These regions are concerned with learning and memory processes, emotion regulation, self-referential processing, and perspective taking.

Precautions, Adverse Effects, and Inclusion of Yoga-Based Meditation for Health, Based on Mind-body Connections

In meditation, particularly open monitor meditation and the *dhyana* state described by Patanjali, meditators are required to engage their attention effortlessly in all aspects of the object of meditation. Because the brain is not actively engaged in a specific activity, there is a possibility that experiences that generally remain unperceived may reach the level of conscious perception.[58] Consequently, patients with posttraumatic stress disorder may experience disturbing memories of trauma or flashbacks. Also, patients whose sense of reality is impaired, such as those with schizophrenia and other psychotic disorders, dissociative disorders, bipolar disorder, or borderline personality, may become more confused and disconnected from reality.[59,60] Hence, meditation is generally not advisable in such conditions. Such patients may benefit more from yoga postures, or certain types of VRYB, and brief guided meditation.

Table 1
Techniques: Method, precautions, and contraindications of voluntarily regulated yoga breathing

I No.	II Category and Name of the Practice	III Technique	IV Precautions and Contraindications Based on Clinical Observations	V Reported Side Effects Based on the Published Literature*
1.	*Change in breath rate: Kapalabhati (HFYB)*	1. Sit erect with backbone and neck in a straight line. 2. Keep your eyes closed. 3. Place a hand on your abdomen and breathe out forcefully through both nostrils, by moving your abdomen/abdominal muscles inward as you breathe out. 4. The rate should not be more than 1 breath/s or 60 breaths/min. 5. After every 3–5 min of practice rest for 1 min. 6. Do not exceed 3 rounds of 5 min per round.	Pregnancy, hypertension, coronary artery disease, recent abdominal/ thoracic surgery, and epilepsy (as it can provoke a seizure). Bipolar disorder, psychosis, history of flashbacks or dissociative, episodes	Single case of pneumothorax following HFYB.[64]
2.	Single nostril breathing	1. Sit erect with your backbone and neck in 1 line. 2. Rest the second and third fingers of your right hand on the bridge of your nose. 3. Gently breathe out through both nostrils. 4. Gently press the outside of the lower right side of the nose with the right thumb, closing the right nostril and breathe in through the left nostril. 5. Breathe out and then in		

| 2a. Alternate nostril yoga breathing | 1. Sit erect with your backbone and neck in 1 line.
2. Rest the second and third fingers of your right hand on the bridge of your nose.
3. Gently breathe out through both nostrils.
4. Gently press the outside of the lower right side of the nose with the right thumb, closing the right nostril and breathe in through the left nostril.
5. Now close the left nostril with the right fourth and fifth fingers and breathe out through the right nostril.
6. Breathe in through the right nostril.
7. Close the right nostril as in step 3. Breathe out through the left nostril and then in through the left nostril. Continue to alternate breathing out and then in through each nostril. | No contraindications | None cited in the literature |
| 2b. Right nostril yoga breathing | 1. Sit erect with your backbone and neck in 1 line.
2. Breathe out through both nostrils.
3. With gentle pressure of the fourth and fifth finger, close the left nostril and breathe in through the right nostril and breathe out through the right nostril. Continue breathing in and out through the right nostril. | Hypertension, anxiety, and insomnia | Prolonged practice can give rise to hypertension in normal individuals (based on findings of increased blood pressure in normal volunteers).[14,16] |

(continued on next page)

Table 1
(continued)

I No.	II Category and Name of the Practice	III Technique	IV Precautions and Contraindications Based on Clinical Observations	V Reported Side Effects Based on the Published Literature*
	2c. Left nostril yoga breathing	1. Sit erect with your backbone and neck in alignment. 2. Breathe out through both nostrils. 3. With gentle pressure of the right thumb, close the right nostril and breathe in through the left nostril and breathe out through the left nostril.	No contraindications	Nil cited in the literature
3.	Breathing with a period of breath-holding (*Kumbhak*)	1. Breath-holding should always be learned in the presence of an experienced instructor. 2. Sit erect with your back and neck in 1 line. 3. Breathe out fully, through the nose. 4. Touch the chin to the chest. 5. Contract the abdominal and perineal muscles completely and in this position hold the breath. 6. Release the chin and relax abdominal and perineal muscles and breathe in.	Contraindications: Pregnancy, hypertension, coronary artery disease, aneurysm, hernia, recent abdominal/thoracic surgery, any abdominal, pelvic, retinal, or pulmonary disease. Bipolar disorder, schizophrenia, dissociative disorder. Adverse effects: dizziness, syncope, stroke.	Nil cited in the literature
	3a. Period of breath-holding shorter than the period of exhalation and inhalation	Ratios 2:1:2:1 where 2 (in):1 (in-hold): 2 (out):1 (out-hold)		
	3b. Period of breath-holding longer than the period of exhalation and inhalation	Ratios 1:4:2:4 using 1 (in):4 (in-hold) : 2 (out):4 (out hold)		

4.	Change in volume of breath: Bellows type breathing with forceful exhalation	1. Sit erect with your spine and neck in 1 line. 2. Breathe in fully and deeply through both nostrils. 3. Breathe out fully through both nostrils. 4. Continue with these deep in and out breaths.	Hypertension, coronary artery disease, recent abdominal/thoracic surgery, and epilepsy.	Nil cited in the literature
5.	Yoga-based meditation techniques			
	5a. Meditative focusing	1. Sit with your spine erect, neck in 1 line, and eyes closed. 2. Normalize your breathing. 3. Make a conscious effort to keep your attention on the object of meditation	Bipolar disorder, psychosis, history of flashbacks or dissociative episodes	Psychosis can be precipitated by meditation in vulnerable persons.[59,60]
	5b. Meditation	1. Sit with your spine erect, neck in the same line, and eyes closed. 2. Normalize your breathing. 3. Allow your awareness to merge with the object of meditation effortlessly.		

Table 2
Clinical outcomes and applications of yoga practices (VRYB and meditation)

I No.	II Technique	III Clinical Outcomes Based on Observation	IV Clinical Outcomes and Applications Based On/ Inferred from Research
1.	Change in breath rate: Kapalabhati (HFYB) (which means "shining forehead" in Sanskrit)	Useful in: 1. Premorbid uncomplicated obesity 2. Learning difficulty 3. Hypersomnia	Useful in: 1. Premorbid uncomplicated obesity.[13] 2. Attention deficit disorder.[18]
2.	Varying the nostril through which one breathes		
	2a. Alternate nostril yoga breathing	1. Lowers blood pressure 2. Increases memory scores, attention, muscle strength, and breath-holding time 3. Rheumatoid arthritis 4. Repetitive stress injury	1. Hypertension.[16] 2. Attention deficit disorder.[17] 3. Spatial memory loss.[20]
	2b. Right nostril yoga breathing	1. Young obese persons	
	2c. Left nostril yoga breathing	1. Anxiety 2. Insomnia	
3.	Breathing with a period of breath holding (Kumbhak, meaning a pot, in Sanskrit)		
	3a. Period of breath holding shorter than the period of exhalation and inhalation	1. Increases energy expenditure 2. Greater arousal	Metabolic syndrome.[11]
	3b. Period of breath holding longer than the period of exhalation and inhalation	1. Lower stress-related arousal 2. Reduction in energy consumption	Lower stress-related arousal.[11]
4.	Change in volume of breath: Bellows-type breathing (Bhastrika, which means bellows in Sanskrit)	1. Reduction in reaction time 2. Improve lung capacity	Better reflex responses.[38]
5.	Yoga-based meditation techniques		
	5a. Meditative focusing	Improved attention	Improved attention.[54]
	5b. Meditation	1. Stress reduction 2. Anxiety	Reduced stress and anxiety.[53]

Despite the precautions mentioned earlier, meditation has a definite place in promoting mental health, preventing mental disorders, and hence, favorably impacting physical health.[61] Accepted concepts of psychoneuroimmunology also suggest applications of meditation in disorders compromising the immune system[62] and in oncology.[63] Details about the method of practice for yoga-based meditation, the precautions and contraindications are provided in **Table 1** and the applications are provided in **Table 2**.

SUMMARY

Ancient yoga texts and present day research explore the linkages between mind and body, including the centrality of breathing. Voluntary regulated breathing techniques provide a conscious way to regulate mental and emotional states. In addition, these techniques have many specific beneficial effects, such as improving attention, memory, reaction time, dexterity, and calmness.

Meditation practices have distinct effects on the endocrine system, the autonomic nervous system, and brain areas, including those involved in attention, executive functions, and emotion regulation. Unstructured meditation is contraindicated in patients with posttraumatic stress disorder who are prone to flashbacks or dissociative episodes, and patients whose sense of reality may be compromised, such as in schizophrenia, bipolar disorder, or borderline personality disorders. Studies are advancing our understanding of the impact of yoga breathing, postures, and meditation on linkages between the mind and the body. Although our scientific knowledge about yoga techniques is growing, further research needs to be undertaken to explore all the potential therapeutic benefits and the underlying mechanism of action for these ancient mind-body practices.

REFERENCES

1. Taimini IK. The science of yoga. Madras (India): The Theosophical Publishing House; 1961.
2. Saraswati S. Asana pranayama mudra bandha. Bihar (India): Yoga Publications Trust; 2006.
3. Vivekananda S. The complete works. Calcutta (India): Advaita Ashrama; 1965.
4. Poon CS. Introduction: optimization hypothesis in the control of breathing. In: Honda Y, Miyamoto Y, Konno K, et al, editors. Control of breathing and its modeling perspective. New York: Plenum; 1992. p. 371–84.
5. Nikhilananda S. The principal Upanishads. New York: Dover Publication Inc; 1975.
6. Gambhirananda S. Taittiriya upanishad. Calcutta (India): Advaita Ashram; 1986.
7. Telles S. A theory of disease from ancient yoga texts. Med Sci Monit 2010;16(6): LE9.
8. Bloch S, Santibáñez HG. Training emotional "effection" in humans: significance of its feedback on subjectivity. In: Bloch S, Aneiros R, editors. Simposio Latinoamericano de Psicobiología del Aprendizaje. Santiago (Chile): Publ. Fac. Med., Universidad de Chile; 1972. p. 170–85.
9. Bloch S, Lemeignan M, Aguilera N. Specific respiratory patterns distinguish among human basic emotions. Int J Psychophysiol 1991;11(2):141–54.
10. Philippot P, Chapelle G, Blairy S. Respiratory feedback in the generation of emotion. Cogn Emot 2002;16(5):605–7.
11. Telles S, Desiraju T. Oxygen consumption during pranayamic type of very slow-rate breathing. Indian J Med Res 1991;94(B):357–63.

12. Telles S, Nagarathna R, Nagendra HR. Breathing through a particular nostril can alter metabolism and autonomic activities. Indian J Physiol Pharmacol 1994; 38(2):133–7.
13. Telles S, Singh N. High frequency yoga breathing increases energy expenditure from carbohydrates. Med Sci Monit 2011;17(9):LE7–8.
14. Telles S, Nagarathna R, Nagendra HR. Physiological measures during right nostril breathing. J Altern Complement Med 1996;2(4):479–84.
15. Bhargava R, Gogate MG, Mascarenhas JF. Autonomic responses to breath holding and its variations following pranayama. Indian J Physiol Pharmacol 1988;32(4):257–64.
16. Raghuraj P, Telles S. Immediate effect of specific nostril manipulating yoga breathing practices on autonomic and respiratory variables. Appl Psychophysiol Biofeedback 2008;33(2):65–75.
17. Telles S, Raghuraj P, Maharana S, et al. Immediate effect of three breathing techniques on performance in a letter cancellation task. Percept Mot Skills 2007; 104(3 Pt 2):1289–96.
18. Telles S, Raghuraj P, Arankalle D, et al. Immediate effect of high-frequency yoga breathing on attention. Indian J Med Sci 2008;62(1):20–2.
19. Shannahoff-Khalsa DS, Boyle MR, Buebel ME. The effects of unilateral forced nostril breathing on cognition. Int J Neurosci 1991;57(3–4):239–49.
20. Naveen KV, Nagarathna R, Nagendra HR, et al. Yoga breathing through a particular nostril increases spatial memory scores without lateralized effects. Psychol Rep 1997;81(2):555–61.
21. Fredrikson M, Engel BT. Cardiovascular and electrodermal adjustments during a vigilance task in patients with borderline and established hypertension. J Psychosom Res 1985;29(3):235–46.
22. Raghuraj P, Ramakrishnan AG, Nagendra HR, et al. Effect of two selected yogic-breathing techniques on heart rate variability. Indian J Physiol Pharmacol 1998; 42(4):467–72.
23. Telles S, Singh N, Balkrishna A. Heart rate variability changes during high frequency yoga breathing and breath awareness. Biopsychosoc Med 2011;5:4.
24. Pramanik T, Pudasaini B, Prajapati R. Immediate effect of a slow pace breathing exercise Bhramari pranayama on blood pressure and heart rate. Nepal Med Coll J 2010;12(3):154–7.
25. Telles S, Nagarathna R, Nagendra HR. Autonomic changes while mentally repeating two syllables – one meaningful and the other neutral. Indian J Physiol Pharmacol 1998;42(1):57–63.
26. Vialatte FB, Bakardjian H, Prasad R, et al. EEG paroxysmal gamma waves during Bhramari Pranayama: a yoga breathing technique. Conscious Cogn 2008;18(4): 977–88.
27. Telles S, Joseph C, Venkatesh S, et al. Alteration of auditory middle latency evoked potentials during yogic consciously regulated breathing and attentive state of mind. Int J Psychophysiol 1992;14(3):189–98.
28. Telles S, Nagarathna R, Nagendra HR, et al. Alterations in auditory middle latency evoked potentials during meditation on a meaningful symbol—'OM'. Int J Neurosci 1994;76(1–2):87–93.
29. Raghuraj P, Telles S. Right uninostril yoga breathing influences ipsilateral components of middle latency auditory evoked potentials. Neurol Sci 2004;25(5):274–80.
30. Joshi M, Telles S. A nonrandomized non-naïve, comparative study of the effects of kapalabhati and breath awareness on event-related potentials in trained yoga practitioners. J Altern Complement Med 2009;15(3):281–5.

31. Telles S, Joshi M, Somvanshi P. Yoga breathing through a particular nostril is associated with contralateral event-related potential changes. Int J Yoga 2012; 5(2):102–7.
32. Lucas SJ, Ainslie PN, Murrell CJ, et al. Effect of age on exercise-induced alterations in cognitive executive function: relationship to cerebral perfusion. Exp Gerontol 2012;47(8):541–51.
33. Ganong WF, Ganong W. Review of medical physiology. New York: McGraw-Hill, Medical York; 2005.
34. Telles S, Singh N, Gupta RK, et al. Optical topography recording of cortical activity during high frequency yoga breathing and breath awareness. Med Sci Monit 2011;17(12):CR692–7.
35. Fuster JM. Executive frontal functions. Exp Brain Res 2000;133:66–70.
36. Telles S, Singh N, Balkrishna A. Finger dexterity and visual discrimination following two yoga breathing practices. Int J Yoga 2011;5(1):37–41.
37. Telles S, Maharana K, Balrana B, et al. Effects of high-frequency yoga breathing called kapalabhati compared with breath awareness on the degree of optical illusion perceived. Percept Mot Skills 2011;112(3):981–90.
38. Bhavanani AB, Madan M, Udupa K. Acute effect of Mukh bhastrika (a yogic bellows type breathing) on reaction time. Indian J Physiol Pharmacol 2003; 47(3):297–300.
39. Telles S, Yadav A, Kumar N, et al. Blood pressure and Purdue pegboard scores in individuals with hypertension after alternate nostril breathing, breath awareness, and no intervention. Med Sci Monit 2013;19:61–6.
40. Miyamura M, Nishimura K, Ishida K, et al. Is man able to breathe once a minute for an hour?: the effect of yoga respiration on blood gases. Jpn J Physiol 2002; 52(3):313–6.
41. Madan M, Jatiya L, Udupa K, et al. Effect of yoga training on hand grip, respiratory pressures and pulmonary function. Indian J Physiol Pharmacol 2003;47(4): 387–92.
42. Jerath R, Edry JW, Barnes VA, et al. Physiology of long pranayamic breathing: neural respiratory elements may provide a mechanism that explains how slow deep breathing shifts the autonomic nervous system. Med Hypotheses 2006; 67(3):566–71.
43. Abelson JL, Khan S, Lyubkin M, et al. Respiratory irregularity and stress hormones in panic disorder: exploring potential linkages. Depress Anxiety 2008;25(10):885–7.
44. Vedamurthachar A, Janakiramaiah N, Hegde JM, et al. Antidepressant efficacy and hormonal effects of Sudarshana Kriya Yoga (SKY) in alcohol dependent individuals. J Affect Disord 2006;94(1–3):249–53.
45. Muktibodhananda S. Hatha yoga pradipika. Bihar (India): Yoga Publication Trust; 2002.
46. Wallace RK. Physiological effects of transcendental meditation. Science 1970; 167(3926):1751–4.
47. Lang R, Dehof K, Meurer KA, et al. Sympathetic activity and transcendental meditation. J Neural Transm 1979;44(1–2):117–35.
48. Corby JC, Roth WT, Zarcone VP Jr, et al. Psychophysiological correlates of the practice of tantric yoga meditation. Arch Gen Psychiatry 1978; 35(5):571.
49. Telles S, Desiraju T. Heart rate and respiratory changes accompanying yogic conditions of single thought and thoughtless states. Indian J Physiol Pharmacol 1992;36(4):293–4.

50. Cahn BR, Polich J. Meditation states and traits: EEG, ERP, and neuroimaging studies. Psychol Bull 2006;132(2):180–211.
51. Telles S, Raghavendra BR, Naveen KV, et al. Changes in autonomic variables following two meditative states described in yoga texts. J Altern Complement Med 2013;19(1):35–42.
52. Kumar S, Nagendra H, Naveen K, et al. Brainstem auditory-evoked potentials in two meditative mental states. Int J Yoga 2010;3(2):37–41.
53. Telles S, Raghavendra BR, Naveen KV. Mid-latency auditory evoked potentials in 2 meditative states. Clin EEG Neurosci 2012;43(2):154–60.
54. Kumar S, Telles S. Meditative states based on yoga texts and their effects on performance of a cancellation task. Percept Mot Skills 2009;109(3):679–89.
55. Streeter CC, Jensen JE, Perlmutter RM, et al. Yoga Asana sessions increase brain GABA levels: a pilot study. J Altern Complement Med 2007;13(4):419–26.
56. Streeter CC, Whitfield TH, Owen L, et al. Effects of yoga versus walking on mood, anxiety, and brain GABA levels: a randomized controlled MRS study. J Altern Complement Med 2010;16(11):1145–52.
57. Hölzel BK, Carmody J, Vangel M, et al. Mindfulness practice leads to increases in regional brain gray matter density. Psychiatry Res 2011;191(1):36–43.
58. Brown DP. A model for the levels of concentrative meditation. Int J Clin Exp Hypn 1977;25(4):236–73.
59. Naveen KV, Telles S. 2009 yoga and psychosis: risks and therapeutic potential. J Indian Psychol 2009;21(1):34–7.
60. Walsh R, Roche L. Precipitation of acute psychotic episodes by intensive meditation in individuals with a history of schizophrenia. Am J Psychiatry 1979;136(8):1085–6.
61. Manocha R, Black D, Wilson L. Quality of life and functional health status of long-term meditators. Evid Based Complement Alternat Med 2012;2012:350674.
62. Jacobs TL, Epel ES, Lin J, et al. Intensive meditation training, immune cell telomerase activity, and psychological mediators. Psychoneuroendocrinology 2011;36(5):664–81.
63. Witek-Janusek L, Albuquerque K, Chroniak KR, et al. Effect of mindfulness based stress reduction on immune function, quality of life and coping in women newly diagnosed with early stage breast cancer. Brain Behav Immun 2008;22(6):969–81.
64. Johnson DB, Tierney MJ, Sadighi PJ. Kapalabhati pranayama: breath of fire or cause of pneumothorax? A case report. Chest 2004;125(5):1951–2.

Tai Chi and Qigong for the Treatment and Prevention of Mental Disorders

Ryan Abbott, MD, JD, MTOM[a], Helen Lavretsky, MD, MS[b],*

KEYWORDS

- Mental health • Quality of life • Nonpharmacologic
- Complementary and alternative medicine • Integrative medicine • Tai Chi • Qigong

KEY POINTS

- Tai Chi and Qigong are evidence-based approaches to improve health-related quality of life, and they may be effective for a range of physical health conditions.
- Evidence from randomized controlled trials suggests that Tai Chi and Qigong may be effective in reducing depressive symptoms, stress, anxiety, and mood disturbances.
- Minimal research supports Tai Chi and Qigong as promising treatments for Parkinson disease, traumatic brain injury, insomnia, substance abuse, and cognitive impairment.
- Indications for Tai Chi and Qigong include inadequate response to other evidence-based treatments, physical comorbidities known to be responsive to Tai Chi and Qigong, patients interested in exercise-based or mindfulness-based interventions, and in geriatric patients who are more susceptible to adverse effects from pharmacologic therapies.

OVERVIEW
Tai Chi and Qigong

Tai Chi and Qigong are traditional Chinese exercises that are widely practiced for their health benefits and as martial arts. Developed over hundreds and thousands of years, respectively, Tai Chi and Qigong are practiced worldwide in a variety of modern and traditional forms. In 2002, there were more than 2.5 million Tai Chi users and

This work was supported by the NIH grants MH077650, MH86481 and AT003480, Forest Research Institute, and Alzheimer's Research and Prevention Foundation to Dr Lavretsky.
^a Southwestern Law School, 3050 Wilshire Boulevard, Los Angeles, California; ^b Department of Psychiatry and Biobehavioral Sciences, Semel Institute for Neuroscience and Human Behavior, David Geffen School of Medicine at UCLA, 760 Westwood Plaza, Los Angeles, CA 90095, USA
* Corresponding author. Department of Psychiatry and Biobehavioral Sciences, Semel Institute for Neuroscience and Human Behavior, David Geffen School of Medicine at UCLA, 760 Westwood Plaza, C9-948A, Los Angeles, CA 90095.
E-mail address: hlavrets@ucla.edu

Psychiatr Clin N Am 36 (2013) 109–119
http://dx.doi.org/10.1016/j.psc.2013.01.011
0193-953X/13/$ – see front matter © 2013 Elsevier Inc. All rights reserved.

500,000 Qigong users in the United States.[1] Both Tai Chi and Qigong involve sequences of flowing movements coupled with changes in mental focus, breathing, coordination, and relaxation.[2] There is significant overlap between the 2 practices in terms of movements and in the shared focus on breathing and mindfulness. Both practices are low-impact, moderate-intensity aerobic exercises that are suitable for a diverse patient population with regards to gender, age, and health status.[3] Tai Chi and Qigong have been characterized as mind-body interventions and as "meditative movements."[4] They are relatively safe, nonpharmacologic practices, which can be used for treatment and prevention of psychosomatic disorders, with few adverse events reported in the literature.[5]

Putative Physiologic Mechanism of Response

Tai Chi and Qigong have been shown to promote relaxation and decrease sympathetic output.[6–9] Relaxation interventions are known to reduce clinical somatic symptoms and to benefit anxiety, depression, blood pressure, and recovery from immune-mediated diseases.[10] Tai Chi and Qigong have been shown to improve immune function and vaccine-response,[11] to increase blood levels of endorphins[12] and baroreflex sensitivity,[13] as well as to reduce levels of inflammatory markers (C-reactive protein [CRP]),[14] adrenocorticotropic hormone,[12] and cortisol.[15,16]

Electroencephalography (EEG) studies of participants undergoing Tai Chi and Qigong exercise have found increased frontal EEG α, β, and θ wave activity, suggesting increased relaxation and attentiveness.[17–19] These changes have not been present in exercise controls.[20,21]

Clinical Research Applications of the Use of Tai Chi and Qigong

A growing body of clinical research has begun to evaluate the efficacy and safety of Tai Chi and Qigong. A systematic review of Tai Chi interventions published in 2011 found 31 Tai Chi randomized controlled trials (RCTs) published from 2002 to 2007, and 11 for 1992 to 2001.[22] That study found suboptimal quality of reporting of Tai Chi intervention trials, with only 23% of RCTs providing adequate details of the Tai Chi intervention used in the trials. Another review of Tai Chi from 1993 to 2007 found 77 RCTs and concluded "research has demonstrated consistent, significant results for many health benefits in RCTs, evidencing progress toward recognizing the similarity and equivalence of Qigong and Tai Chi." The study found 6410 participants included across these reported studies.

Problematic research issues within the literature on Tai Chi and Qigong are usually related to small sample size, use of different styles of Tai Chi and Qigong, significant variance in practice duration and frequency, and differences in study durations. Because of the similarity of Tai Chi and Qigong and because clinical research has largely failed to differentiate between the 2 exercises, this review considers the benefits of both practices.[23]

Health Outcomes of Tai Chi and Qigong Interventions

RCTs have shown that Tai Chi and Qigong may improve bone density, cardiopulmonary health, arthritis, fibromyalgia, tension headaches, and other medical conditions.[24–36]

Given the relationship between physical and mental health, general improvements in physical health or reductions of chronic disease symptoms may help to improve mental health. Chronic physical health problems are associated with stress, anxiety, depression, and poor mood.[37,38]

Health-Related Quality of Life

Health-related quality of life (HRQOL) serves as a comprehensive measure of patient well-being, and it reflects patient perceptions of personal health and life satisfaction over a period of time. Individuals suffering from mental health conditions are particularly likely to report poor HRQOL. A study comparing patients with common medical disorders to those with mental health conditions found significant differences in HRQOL between the 2 groups. Individuals with mental health conditions had significantly greater impairment of HRQOL.[39] The ability of Tai Chi and Qigong to improve HRQOL[31,40,41] is an important consideration for treating patients with mental disorders. Although there is no evidence that Tai Chi and Qigong may be effective for a particular condition, they may still provide some benefit by improving HRQOL.

Tai Chi and Qigong as Exercise

Studies have tried to understand the effects of Tai Chi and Qigong as aerobic versus mindful exercise. Independent from any special benefits Tai Chi and Qigong may confer as meditative movements, they also benefit patients as general, low-impact, moderate-intensity aerobic exercise. There is extensive evidence on general exercise interventions with regards to mental disorders.[42] Systematic reviews have found that exercise results in significant reductions in depression symptoms comparable with cognitive-behavioral therapy.[43,44] Two studies found that exercise is comparable with sertraline (Zoloft) in terms of efficacy for treatment of major depressive disorder. In studies comparing the benefits of Tai Chi and Qigong with general exercise, both interventions have been shown to have comparable effects at reducing anxiety.[45,46] In general, evidence from clinical trials supports a positive association between physical activity and physical and psychological health.[47–50]

Tai Chi and Qigong as Meditative Practices

Tai Chi and Qigong practices include a mindfulness component, which may explain why some patients experience greater benefits from Tai Chi or Qigong than from general aerobic exercises.[16,46] A Cochrane collaboration review of meditation therapy for anxiety disorders found only a few studies that permitted firm conclusions on efficacy. The review identified 50 studies of meditation on anxiety, but only 2 that were randomized, controlled and that met criteria for *Diagnostic and Statistical Manual of Mental Disorders* or *International Classification of Diseases* classification of a psychiatric disorder. These 2 studies were of moderate quality with active control comparisons (alternative meditation, biofeedback, or relaxation). One of these studies, which used transcendental meditation, showed a reduction in anxiety and electromyography score comparable with biofeedback and relaxation therapy.[51] The other study compared Kundalini yoga with relaxation/mindfulness meditation and found no significant difference between groups. A separate review concluded that several studies of exercise and yoga have shown benefits comparable with established depression and anxiety treatments. A third review compared 12 RCTs of mindfulness exercises versus nonmindfulness exercises and found that both were effective in causing short-term reductions in depression levels and symptoms.[49]

An RCT of brief daily yogic meditation (Kirtan Kriya) for family dementia caregivers with mild depressive symptoms found that meditation resulted in lower levels of depressive symptoms as well as improvements in mental health and cognitive functioning. Participants in the yogic meditation group showed a 43% improvement in telomerase activity after 12 minutes of daily practice for 8 weeks, compared with 3.7% in relaxation music control participants. This finding suggests that brief daily meditation practices may lead to improved mental and cognitive functioning and may also benefit stress-induced cellular aging. Another report found that Kirtan Kriya reversed the pattern of increased nuclear factor κB (NF-κB)-related transcription of proinflammatory cytokines and decreased interferon regulatory factor 1–related transcription of innate antiviral response genes in distressed dementia caregivers. This finding reinforces the relationship between stress reduction and beneficial immune response.[52]

RESEARCH APPLICATIONS TO MENTAL HEALTH
Psychosocial Well-Being

The evidence base for Tai Chi on psychosocial well-being was evaluated in a meta-analysis published in 2010[53] and a systematic review published in 2009.[54] The meta-analysis identified 40 studies (17 RCTs, 16 nonrandomized comparison studies [NRSs], and 7 observational studies) with a total of 3817 individuals reporting at least 1 psychological health outcome from a search of 11 English and Chinese databases. Twenty-one of the 33 RCTs and NRSs found that in community-dwelling participants between 1 hour up to 1 year of regular Tai Chi significantly increased psychological well-being, reduced stress (effect size [ES], 0.66; 95% confidence interval [CI], 0.23–1.09), anxiety (ES, 0.66; 95% CI, 0.29–1.03), and depression (ES, 0.56; 95% CI, 0.31–0.80), and enhanced mood (ES, 0.45; 95% CI, 0.20–0.69).

The review concluded that "Tai Chi appears to be associated with improvements in psychological well-being including reduced stress, anxiety, depression and mood disturbance, and increased self-esteem. Definitive conclusions were limited due to variation in designs, comparisons, heterogeneous outcomes, and inadequate controls. High-quality, well-controlled, longer randomized trials are needed to better inform clinical decisions."[53] This systematic review limited analysis to 15 RCTs published in English because of concerns about study quality in the non-English literature. The reviewers identified a subset of 8 high-quality trials that together included evaluations of anxiety, depression, mood, stress, general mental health, anger, positive and negative effect, self-esteem, life satisfaction, social interaction, and self-rated health. Tai Chi was found to have a significant positive effect in 13 of the 15 studies, and in 6 of the 8 high-quality trials. Earlier reviews have concluded that Tai Chi seems to improve psychosocial well-being.[55–57]

The effects of Tai Chi on self-esteem have been evaluated in 3 RCTs.[58] All of these studies found an increase in self-esteem compared with control groups, but only 1 produced statistically significant between-group results.[58] That study randomized 21 women diagnosed with breast cancer who had completed treatment within the last 30 months to receive 12 weeks of Tai Chi or psychosocial support 3 times a week. A review of 51 studies of general exercise found that aerobic exercise is effective in improving self-esteem.[59]

Stress Management

The most logical clinical application of mind-body techniques is for stress reduction. Out of 5 RCTs, 4 found a significant association between Tai Chi and Qigong and positive effects on stress.

1. Beneficial effects were found in a study in 2008[60] that evaluated a population infected with the human immunodeficiency virus (mean age 42 years, n = 252) randomized to practice Tai Chi for 90 minutes once weekly for 10 weeks or to a cognitive-behavioral relaxation group, spiritual growth group, or a wait-list control group.

2. A study in 2001[61] that used a healthy geriatric population (mean age 73 years, n = 72) randomized to practice Tai Chi for 1 hour twice weekly for 24 weeks versus a wait-list control group also found that Tai Chi reduced stress.
3. Tai Chi was shown to reduce stress in a study in 1996[62] that evaluated health among older adults (mean age 67 years, n = 20) who practiced Tai Chi for 2 hours, once weekly for 10 sessions compared with a routine physical activity group.
4. Positive effects were found in a study in 1992[45] that looked at healthy adults (mean age 36 years, n = 96) who underwent a single, 1-hour session of Tai Chi versus meditation, brisk walking, or neutral reading.
5. One RCT did not find positive results; a study in 2007[63] that evaluated individuals with hip or knee osteoarthritis (mean age 70 years, n = 152) who practiced Tai Chi for an hour twice weekly for 12 weeks found no significant difference compared with a hydrotherapy or wait-list control group.

All studies used subjective stress measures, 1 measured body temperature,[62] and 2 measured salivary cortisol levels,[60] which decreased as a result of Tai Chi practice.

Mood, Anxiety, and Depression

Seven RCTs have found that Tai Chi significantly improves mood, including:

- A 2011 study of 100 outpatients (mean age 67 years) with systolic heart failure who received either a 12-week Tai Chi exercise program or time-matched education.
- A study published in 2009 randomized 21 obese women to either a 2-hour weekly session of Tai Chi or a conventional structured exercise program and found that only the Tai Chi group experienced improvements in mood.
- Benefits to mood were also found in a 2005 study of 38 adults (20–60 years old) with advanced HIV/AIDS who participated in 8 weeks of twice weekly, 1-hour-long Tai Chi practice versus aerobic exercise or usual activity.[64]
- A 1995 study of 135 healthy, sedentary adults (mean age 53 years) who practiced Tai Chi for 45 minutes, 3 times a week, for 16 weeks reported improved mood compared with exercise and relaxation control groups.[65]
- Three of the trials described earlier[45,60,61] also found benefits to mood.

An RCT[66] found no significant impact of Tai Chi on mood. That trial randomized 22 community-dwelling participants (mean age 68 years) with lower extremity osteoarthritis to 12 weeks of twice-weekly, 1-hour-long Tai Chi sessions or to a control group. Tai Chi was found to improve pain, physical function, and other arthritis symptoms (measured using the Arthritis Self-Efficacy Scale) as well as satisfaction with general health status, but it did not result in a statistically significant difference in mood.

Ten RCTs have investigated the effects of Tai Chi on anxiety, 9 of which showed significant positive effects.

- A Japanese trial in 2010[67] evaluated 34 community-dwelling elderly participants with cerebral vascular disorder who were randomized to receive either Tai Chi or standard rehabilitation in group sessions once weekly for 12 weeks. Participants in the Tai Chi group experienced improvements in sleep quality, anxiety/insomnia, and depression.
- A study in 2008[33] randomized 20 patients with rheumatoid arthritis to 12 weeks of twice-weekly sessions of Tai Chi or attention control. Participants in the Tai Chi group experienced greater improvements in anxiety and depression than the control group.

- A study in 2007[35] of 65 patients (mean age 70 years) with chronic heart failure received 16 weeks of either Tai Chi practice twice weekly or standard medical care without exercise rehabilitation. They reported that both groups had a significant reduction in anxiety scores, found no between-group differences in anxiety, and found that depression was reduced only in the Tai Chi group.
- A study in 2007[68] of 84 sedentary older people (mean age 70 years) contrasted Tai Chi with low-impact exercise for 12 weeks and found that both groups of patients experienced improvements in anxiety.
- A study in 2003[69] of 76 healthy individuals (mean age 52 years) found improvements in anxiety for participants who received 12 weeks of 50-minute Tai Chi sessions 3 times a week compared with a sedentary life control group.
- Improvements to anxiety were also found in 3 RCTs described earlier.[45]
- One RCT described earlier[63] did not find a significant effect on anxiety.

Fourteen RCTs have evaluated the effects of Tai Chi and Qigong on depressive symptoms, 13 of which found positive results. Several of these RCTs have already been described.[67]

- A single-blind, 12-week study[70] of participants with fibromyalgia (mean age 50 years, n = 66) published in 2009 found that Tai Chi produced greater improvements in depression than a stretching and wellness education group.
- Another single-blind, 12-week trial in 2009[71] randomized 40 patients (mean age 65 years) with knee osteoarthritis to receive either Tai Chi or wellness education and stretching and found that patients in the Tai Chi group experienced greater improvement in depression.
- An RCT in 2008 evaluated 14 community-dwelling older patients from a psychogeriatric outpatient clinic who were randomized to receive a 3-month Tai Chi intervention or to a wait-list control. Only the Tai Chi group experienced improvements in depressive symptoms.
- A trial in 2007 randomized 112 healthy older adults (aged 59–86 years) to 25 weeks of either Tai Chi or health education. Participants in both groups experienced improvements in depressive symptoms.
- An RCT in 2005[72] of 291 women and 20 men (aged 70–97 years) recruited from 10 matched pairs of congregate living facilities found that 48 weeks of Tai Chi led to a significantly greater reduction in depression than wellness education ($P < 0.001$).
- A Chinese trial in 2004[21] randomized 14 elderly persons (mean age 73 years) with depression to 12 weeks of Tai Chi 3 times a week for 45 minutes or to a wait-list control group. Only the Tai Chi group experienced improvements in depressive symptoms.
- A trial in 1998[73] of 51 patients aged 18 to 60 years with chronic low back pain reported improvements in depressive symptoms compared with a control group after 6 weeks practicing Tai Chi once a week for 90 minutes.
- Only 1 RCT did not find evidence that Tai Chi and Qigong are effective in reducing depressive symptoms or had any effect on anxiety or stress management.[63]

Most of these studies were conducted in patient populations without known mental disorders. Only 2 studies involved participants with clinically diagnosed depression.[72] A review in 2009[74] of Tai Chi and Qigong in older adults found 36 clinical trials with 3799 participants and concluded that Tai Chi and Qigong practice causes significant improvement in depression and anxiety. Tai Chi has been particularly recommended as a first-line treatment of mild depression in geriatric populations given its known benefits in improving balance and reducing falls.[75] Depression and falls are associated through a complex bidirectional relationship.[76] Antidepressant use has also been associated with falls,[77] especially selective serotonin reuptake inhibitors, which are associated with fragility fractures to a higher degree than other classes of psychotropic medications.[78,79]

On the other hand, more recent research has produced mixed results on the effectiveness of Tai Chi and Qigong for prevention of falls. One Cochrane collaboration meta-analysis[80] found that Tai Chi had a moderate effect on reducing falls in community-based geriatric populations, and a second meta-analysis[81] found insufficient evidence to support the use of Tai Chi for prevention of falls. One of the most recent RCTs of Tai Chi as a community-based falls prevention intervention was an 11-site multicenter study conducted in New Zealand.[82] A total of 684 community-residing older adults with at least 1 risk factor for falls were randomized to receive 20 weeks of either Tai Chi once a week, Tai Chi twice a week, or general exercise once a week. All groups experienced a reduction in rate of falls; however, there was no statistically significant difference between groups over the 17-month follow-up period.

Sleep Disturbance

Tai Chi and Qigong may also be able to improve sleep quality, with corresponding impact on mental health.

- An RCT[6] of Tai Chi for improving sleep quality in older adults with moderate sleep complaints randomized[67] 112 participants to receive 25 weeks of either Tai Chi or health education. The study found that participants in the Tai Chi group were more likely to achieve a treatment response and to show global improvements in sleep quality.
- A second RCT[83] in a geriatric (aged 60–92 years) population (n = 118) found that Tai Chi, practiced for an hour, 3 times weekly for 24 weeks, was more effective than general exercise at improving sleep quality and daytime sleepiness.
- A third RCT,[67] described earlier, found that 12 weeks of Tai Chi practice once a week was more effective at improving sleep quality than a rehabilitation control group. Chronic sleep problems are associated with impaired health status and depressive symptoms.[84]
- A fourth RCT[85] assigned 102 community-dwelling participants (mean age 68.9 years) in Vietnam to receive 6 months of Tai Chi training or to maintain their routine daily activities. Compared with the control group, individuals in the Tai Chi group experienced significant improvements in sleep quality, balance, and cognitive performance.

Substance Abuse

A Chinese RCT[86] of 86 patients randomized to a Qigong treatment group, medication group, or no-treatment control group reported that participants in the Qigong group experienced comparatively fewer withdrawal symptoms. Qigong was also credited with a lower relapse rate and improved anxiety scores. A nonrandomized controlled trial of 248 patients in a short-term residential treatment program who self-selected participation in either a Qigong meditation program or stress management plus relaxation program reported that Qigong participants experienced a higher treatment completion rate and greater reduction in cravings.[87] Participants were offered Qigong meditation twice daily, 5 or more days a week, for a total of 2 weeks. The study noted that female Qigong participants reported significantly more reduction in anxiety and withdrawal than any other group.

Cognitive Functioning

Published interim results from a year-long Chinese RCT[88] suggest that Tai Chi may provide a cognitive benefit. The study randomized 389 geriatric participants with dementia or amnestic mild cognitive impairment to either a Tai Chi group or a strengthening and toning exercise group. After 5 months of triweekly practice sessions, both groups showed improvements in global cognitive function, delayed recall, and subjective complaints. Only the Tai Chi group maintained a stable clinical dementia rating and showed improvements in visual spans.

Another RCT of healthy community-dwelling older adults (mean age 69 years, n = 132) found that Tai Chi produced greater improvements in a cognitive function measure than a Western exercise or attention control group. The improvement in cognitive functioning was maintained throughout the 12-month follow-up period. An RCT described earlier found that Tai Chi improves motor speed and visual attention in elderly individuals.

Parkinson Disease

An RCT in 2012[89] of 195 patients found that 24 weeks of Tai Chi was more effective than resistance training or stretching at improving primary balance outcomes (maximum excursion and directional control). The Tai Chi group also performed better than the stretching group in all secondary balance measures, including strength, functional reach, timed up-and-go tests, motor scores, and number of falls. The Tai Chi group performed better than the resistance group in stride length and functional reach. The effects of Tai Chi training were maintained 3 months after the end of the intervention, and no serious adverse events were observed. The study concluded that Tai Chi seems to reduce balance impairments in patients with mild-to-moderate Parkinson disease, with the additional benefits of improving functional capacity and reducing falls.

Other trials of Tai Chi and Qigong in populations with Parkinson disease have found similar results. An RCT in 2008 (n = 33) found that 20, 1-hour sessions of Tai Chi were effective at improving several balance measures, and at improving well-being compared with a no-intervention control group.[90] Another RCT (n = 30) found that a 12-week Tai Chi program was effective in reducing falls and slowing functional decline.

Traumatic Brain Injury

With the increased interest in traumatic brain injury (TBI), an RCT of 20 patients with TBI found that participation in Qigong improved mood and self-esteem relative to a nonexercise control group, but it found no difference in physical functioning between groups. Participants in that study attended a Qigong exercise session for 1 hour per week over 8 weeks, whereas control participants engaged in non–exercise-based social and leisure activities. A second RCT[91] evaluated 18 participants with TBI assigned to either a wait-list control or Tai Chi group and found that Tai Chi provided short-term benefits after TBI. The participants in the 6-week Tai Chi course had improved outcomes in HRQOL, self-esteem, and mood. Patients with TBI often suffer from cognitive, emotional, and mental challenges.[92]

See **Table 1** for a summary of RCTs of Tai Chi and Qigong for mental disorders.

SUMMARY/DISCUSSION
Complementary Approaches to Pharmacologic Strategies

Tai Chi and Qigong are nonpharmacologic treatments that can be used in conjunction with pharmacologic treatments. Nonpharmacologic approaches to mental disorders

Table 1
The summary of the RCTs of Tai Chi and Qigong for mental disorders

	Positive Findings	Negative Findings
Depression	Thirteen studies with significant positive findings,[11,21,33,34,61,63,65–73,93]; only 2 with clinically diagnosed depression populations[21,72]	One study did not find effect on depressive symptoms[63]
Stress	Four studies with significant positive findings,[60] subjective stress measures,[45,60–63] body temperature,[62] and salivary cortisol levels[45,60]	One study did not find effect on subjective stress measures[63]
Anxiety	Eight studies with significant positive effects[67]	One study had negative findings on anxiety[35,63]
Mood and psychological well-being	Seven studies with significant positive effects[93,94]	One study did not find positive effect on mood[66]
Self-esteem	One study with significant positive effects[58]	Two without positive effect[65,95]
Parkinson disease	Three studies with significant positive effects[89,90,96]	
TBI	Two studies with significant positive effects[91,97]	None reported
Sleep disturbance	Three studies with significant positive effects[67,83,91]	None reported
Substance abuse	One study with significant positive effects[86]	None reported
Cognitive functioning	Two studies with significant positive effects[88,98]	None reported

are particularly important given that many patients fail to achieve symptomatic remission and functional recovery with first-line pharmacotherapy.[99,100] Treatments are needed to complement pharmacotherapies to help patients achieve remission, experience reductions in mental disorder symptoms, and enjoy improved social and health functioning.[101]

Limited research has specifically evaluated Tai Chi and Qigong as a combined treatment with pharmaceutical intervention. A study of older adults with major depression found that the complementary use of Tai Chi augments the use of escitalopram (Lexapro). The study randomized 73 partial responders to escitalopram, who continued to use escitalopram daily, to a 10-week course of either Tai Chi or health education. Individuals in the Tai Chi group were more likely to report greater reduction in depressive symptoms and to achieve a depression remission ($F_{[5, 285]} = 2.26$; $P<.05$). Those individuals also showed greater improvements in HRQOL physical functioning (group $\times$ time interaction: $F_{[1, 66]} = 5.73$; $P = .02$) and cognition (ie, memory; group $\times$ time interaction: $F_{[1, 65]} = 5.29$; $P<.05$), and a decline in an inflammatory marker, CRP (time effect: $F_{[2, 78]} = 3.14$, $P<.05$ and group $\times$ time trend in posttreatment period: $F_{[1, 39]} = 2.91$; $P = .10$).[14]

Clinical Recommendations

There is not strong evidence that Tai Chi and Qigong are effective as either primary or complementary treatments for mental disorders. Only a few mental and neurologic disorders have been specifically evaluated in the literature. As the evidence for Tai Chi and Qigong continues to develop, promising results from multiple RCTs suggest that these are potentially effective treatments for reducing stress, anxiety, depression, and low mood, as well as for improving self-esteem and general psychosocial well-being. Results from the RCTs evaluating Tai Chi and Qigong for specific mental diseases suggest that they may be effective for improving symptoms of Parkinson disease, TBI, sleep disturbance, substance abuse, and cognitive impairment. There remains a pressing need for methodologically robust studies of Tai Chi and Qigong for mental disorders. Multiple RCTs may have produced mixed results on the efficacy of Tai Chi and Qigong for a particular indication because of the variations in designs, comparisons, patient populations, and interventions.[54] Few studies evaluated patient populations with diagnosed mental disorders.

Given that Tai Chi and Qigong are nonpharmacologic and noninvasive treatments, recommending these exercises to patients with mental disorders generally seems an appropriate option for clinicians, particularly for conditions that have been studied in RCTs. Whether or not Tai Chi and Qigong can improve disease-specific outcomes, significant evidence supports the assertion that Tai Chi and Qigong can improve HRQOL and mental health. Tai Chi and Qigong may be particularly appropriate for patients who have physical comorbidity known to be responsive to Tai Chi and Qigong practice, in geriatric populations, who are more susceptible to adverse effects from pharmacologic therapies, or in patients who choose to use exercise or mind-body practices.

Instructor quality may affect patient outcomes, but this has not been addressed in clinical research. There is no licensing body that regulates Tai Chi teachers and no certifying body that clearly distinguishes higher-quality instructors. Consumers in this market rely largely on word of mouth and local reputation. Although Tai Chi has traditionally been taught 1-on-1 or in class settings, a variety of home exercise programs are publically available for patients who are logistically or financially unable to study in person or who prefer to study independently. For example, Beachbody, LLC (Santa Monica, California), makers of the popular home exercise program *P90X*, sell a home DVD exercise Tai Chi program, *Tai Cheng*.

Practice style, frequency, and duration have been variable. The predominant style of Tai Chi used in the RCTs evaluated in this review was the Yang style or Yang style short-form. Most styles are similar in practice although it is frequently claimed by practitioners that one style is superior. It is unclear that there is any benefit from one style versus another at this point. Regardless of the form of Tai Chi being evaluated, most studies had participants practicing 30 minutes to 2 hours, 1 to 3 times per week. Clinicians prescribing Tai Chi should consider recommending that patients practice for a minimum of 30 minutes, 3 times a week on an ongoing basis. Alternatively, those recommendations may be left to an experienced instructor. Practice durations in the literature are generally in the range of a few weeks to a few months, although studies found both short-term benefits from as little as 1 practice session and long-term benefits in multiyear practitioners. Comparative effectiveness research has not yet addressed the optimal duration of the exercise.

APPENDIX: REFERENCES

The complete reference list is online at http://www.psych.theclinics.com/dx.doi.org/10.1016/j.psc.2013.01.011.

KEY REFERENCES

14. Lavretsky H, Alstein LL, Olmstead RE, et al. Complementary use of tai chi chih augments escitalopram treatment of geriatric depression: a randomized controlled trial. Am J Geriatr Psychiatry 2011;19(10):839–50.

22. Li JY, Zhang YF, Smith GS, et al. Quality of reporting of randomized clinical trials in tai chi interventions–a systematic review. Evid Based Complement Alternat Med 2011;2011:383245.

23. Jahnke R, Larkey L, Rogers C, et al. A comprehensive review of health benefits of qigong and tai chi. Am J Health Promot 2010;24(6):e1–25.

53. Wang C, Bannuru R, Ramel J, et al. Tai Chi on psychological well-being: systematic review and meta-analysis. BMC Complement Altern Med 2010;10:23.

54. Wang WC, Zhang AL, Rasmussen B, et al. The effect of Tai Chi on psychosocial well-being: a systematic review of randomized controlled trials. J Acupunct Meridian Stud 2009;2(3):171–81.

56. Wang C, Collet JP, Lau J. The effect of Tai Chi on health outcomes in patients with chronic conditions: a systematic review. Arch Intern Med 2004; 164(15006825):493–501.

89. Li F, Harmer P, Fitzgerald K, et al. Tai chi and postural stability in patients with Parkinson's disease. N Engl J Med 2012;366(6):511–9.

Breathing Practices for Treatment of Psychiatric and Stress-Related Medical Conditions

Richard P. Brown, MD[a], Patricia L. Gerbarg, MD[b,*],
Fred Muench, PhD[c]

KEYWORDS

- Paced breathing • Pranayama • Resonance breathing • Coherent breathing • Yoga
- Qigong • Anxiety • Depression

KEY POINTS

- Neuroanatomic and brain imaging studies reveal breath-activated pathways to all major networks involved in emotion regulation, cognitive function, attention, perception, subjective awareness, and decision making.
- Specific breath practices have been shown to be beneficial in reducing symptoms of stress, anxiety, insomnia, posttraumatic stress disorder, obsessive-compulsive disorder, depression, attention deficit disorder, and schizophrenia.
- The risks of adverse reactions to breath practices can be minimized through patient assessment and by limiting the use of stimulating practices in vulnerable individuals.
- Technology-assisted breath retraining devices range from mobile phone pacing applications to physiologic biofeedback machines designed to foster therapeutic breath practices using audiovisual cues and/or physiologic feedback.
- Technology-assisted breath retraining offers alternative or adjunctive methods to clients who are interested in breathing practices.
- Ideally, initial technology-assisted breath retraining should be accompanied by in-person guided instruction and evaluation.

INTRODUCTION

Research on breathing techniques is generating new treatments for stress reduction, anxiety disorders, depression, posttraumatic stress disorder (PTSD), attention-deficit

---

Disclosures: R.P. Brown and P.L. Gerbarg: codeveloped the Breath-Body-Mind program and sometimes receive financial remuneration for teaching it; F. Muench: Dr Muench codeveloped the iPhone application, BreathPacer, but as of 2013 no longer receives royalties from the company marketing it.
[a] Department of Psychiatry, Columbia University College of Physicians and Surgeons, 86 Sherry Lane, New York, NY 12401, USA; [b] Department of Psychiatry, New York Medical College, 86 Sherry Lane, Valhalla, NY 12401, USA; [c] Columbia University College of Physicians and Surgeons, 3 Columbus Circle, Suite 1404, New York, NY 10017, USA
* Corresponding author.
E-mail address: PGerbarg@aol.com

Psychiatr Clin N Am 36 (2013) 121–140
http://dx.doi.org/10.1016/j.psc.2013.01.001

disorder, and stress-related medical conditions. Breathing practices can ameliorate aberrations in sympatho-vagal balance, stress response, emotion regulation, and neuroendocrine function associated with these conditions. The first part of this article describes evidence-based breath practices for mental health care; the second part reviews technology-assisted breathing interventions. For each technique, the research support, clinical applications, and the risks and benefits are discussed.

BREATHING PRACTICES: DEFINITIONS AND CONTEXTS

Breathing practices entail voluntary changes in the rate, pattern, and quality of respiration. Many Eastern traditions consider breath practices to be fundamental to physical, emotional, and spiritual development (see article in this publication by *Telles and Singh*). Until recently, the centrality of breath work had been largely lost in transition from East to West. Each practice has innumerable variations, producing different psychophysiological effects.[1,2] The terms *yoga* or *yogic* breathing are used to encompass all of the forms described throughout this discussion.

- *Paced breathing* requires controlling the respiratory rate and the relative length of 4 phases of the breath cycle.
- In *coherent* or *resonance* breathing, the length of inhalation and exhalation are equal with only a slight pause between. Other forms use counts, for example, 4 counts in, 4 counts breath hold, 6 counts out, and 2 counts breath hold.
- *Resistance breathing* creates partial obstruction to airflow using laryngeal contracture, vocal cords, pursed lips, or other means, which produces sounds and vibrations.
- *Unilateral* or *alternate nostril breathing* involves closing one nostril such that all air flows through the other.
- *Moving the breath* engages the imagination to move one's breath through different parts of the body.
- *Breathing with movement* coordinates paced breathing with physical movements.

Yoga styles vary in their emphasis on breathing, movement, and meditation. Iyengar yoga focuses on body alignment with breath practices, Vinyasa on breath-linked movement,[3] and Shavasana on relaxation and rhythmic breathing. Sudarshan Kriya yoga (SKY) includes 5 breath practices:

1. Resistance breath (*Ujjayi*)
2. *Om* chant
3. Bellows breath (*Bhastrika*)
4. Sudarshan Kriya (SK) cyclical breathing at varying rates
5. Alternate nostril breathing (ANB)

Qigong and Tai Chi entail body movements, breath exercises, and meditation to circulate vital energy (*Qi* or *Chi*). Breath-body-mind, a modern adaptation, combines coherent breathing, resistance breathing and breath moving (a qigong meditative practice most highly developed by eleventh century Russian Orthodox Christian monks).[4] Thich Nhat Hanh (2009) allows the breath to slow down naturally by placing awareness on the breath during meditation. Theravadin Buddhism emphasizes meditative breathing, such as anapanasati.[5] Tibetan Buddhist breath practices are considered to be so sacred that they are rarely seen in the West.

PUTATIVE PHYSIOLOGIC MECHANISMS OF ACTION

An evolving neurophysiological model for the effects of breath practices has been described previously.[6–8] Research demonstrates that yoga breathing can modulate autonomic nervous system (ANS) function, stress responses, cardiac vagal tone, heart rate variability (HRV), vigilance, attention, chemoreflex and baroreflex sensitivity, central nervous system excitation, and neuroendocrine functions.[9] Slow breathing at 4.5 to 6.5 breaths per minute (coherent or resonance breathing) has been shown to optimally balance sympatho-vagal stress response for most adults.[10–13]

Imbalances of the ANS, including decreased parasympathetic nervous system (PNS) activity and increased sympathetic nervous system (SNS) activity, underactivity of the inhibitory neurotransmitter, gamma amino-butyric acid (GABA), and increased allostatic load (the cost to the organism to adapt to conditions outside the usual homeostatic range) are associated with depression, anxiety, PTSD, and other psychiatric disorders. These conditions are exacerbated by stress and are characterized by low PNS and low GABA activity. Streeter and colleagues[8] hypothesized that yoga practices are associated with the following effects:

1. Correction of the underactivity of the PNS and GABA system in part through stimulation of the vagal nerves, the main pathway of the PNS
2. Reduction of allostatic load resulting in symptom relief

The om chant involves slow breathing, airway resistance (contracting the vocal cords to generate sound), and vibrational effects, which increase vagal tone and physiologic relaxation.[14] A functional magnetic resonance imaging study showed significant limbic system deactivation with om chanting.[15]

Stress and PTSD are associated with decreased hippocampal GABA levels, prefrontal cortex (PFC) underactivity, amygdalar overactivity, and low HRV.[6,8] Because the underactive PFC fails to inhibit the overactive amygdala (as in PTSD), emotions become dysregulated and limbic defensive reactions emerge. The insular cortex in the sylvian fissure between the temporal and frontal lobes also sends inhibitory GABAergic projections to the central extended amygdala. **Fig. 1** shows neural circuits and anatomic structures with GABA receptors that are hypothesized to regulate stress response systems. It has been proposed that *interoceptive* information (sensory information from inside the body) may be conveyed by the PNS via the *nucleus tractus solitarius* to the insular cortex creating a map of the internal state of the body that may be the substrate for perception and subjective experience of the inside of the body.[16] Changes in breathing patterns alter the interoceptive messages from the body traveling primarily through the vagus nerves to critical regulatory brain centers. When millions of sensors throughout the respiratory system (nose, throat, lungs, bronchial tree, diaphragm, and thorax) send signals, the brain responds with rapid and widespread shifts in activation, attention, perception, emotion regulation, subjective experience, and behavior.[8,9]

Theoretically, yoga breathing stimulates an underactive PNS, increasing the inhibitory action of a hypoactive GABA system in brain pathways and structures that are critical for threat perception, emotion regulation, and stress reactivity. Increased inhibitory GABA transmission from the PFC and/or the insular cortex could reduce overactivity in the amygdala and the associated psychological and somatic symptoms of PTSD (see **Fig. 1**).[8] Vagal pathways to the central PNS also lead to the anterior cingulate,[16] which is involved in evaluation, decision making, emotion regulation, fear extinction, and inhibition of amygdalar reactivity.[17] The hypothalamic-pituitary-adrenal axis is also influenced by the PNS via connections with the hypothalamus,

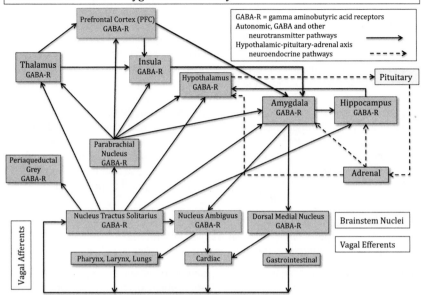

Fig. 1. Neuroanatomic connections of parasympathetic nervous system with GABA system. (*From* Streeter CC, Gerbarg PL, Saper RB, et al. Effects of yoga on the autonomic nervous system, gamma-aminobutyric-acid, and allostasis in epilepsy, depression, and post-traumatic stress disorder. Medical Hypotheses 2012;78(5):571–9; with permission.)

amygdala, and hippocampus (see **Fig. 1**). Yoga practices are associated with reduced levels of stress markers, including cortisol.[18,19] Evidence suggests that vagal activation also increases the release of prosocial hormones, oxytocin, vasopressin, and prolactin, which may contribute to the increase in feelings of love, bonding, empathy, and meaning reported by many yoga practitioners.[20] Breath practices can affect key anatomic structures and neural pathways involved in the regulation of emotion, attention, perception, and problem solving.

SELECTED STUDIES OF BREATH PRACTICES FOR PSYCHIATRIC CONDITIONS

Yoga and other mind-body traditions use movement, breathing, meditation, and other practices. This review includes open and controlled trials of breath practices alone and multicomponent interventions that emphasize breath practices.[3]

Stress Management

Four randomized controlled trials (RCTs) and one open study of slow-paced breathing show reduction in symptoms of stress, anxiety, anger, exhaustion, depression, and improvement in quality of life associated with increased HRV, indicating activation of vagal PNS pathways (**Table 1**).[18,21–24]

Anxiety Disorders, Generalized Anxiety Disorder, Insomnia

Seven studies, including 2 RCTs, 2 controlled trials (CTs), and 3 open pilots, found significant reductions in anxiety with breath-focused yoga programs (see **Table 1**).[25–31]

Generalized anxiety disorder

Two pilot studies evaluated yoga programs for severe treatment-resistant generalized anxiety disorder with comorbidities. In the first study (n = 31) using the 22-hour SKY program, the response rate was 73% and the remission rate was 41%.[25] The second study (n = 20) using the breath-body-mind 12-hour program of breath practices, qigong, and open focus meditation[32] resulted in significant improvements in anxiety, sleep, and depression.[26]

PTSD

Studies of yoga programs emphasizing breath practices for PTSD (3 RCTs, one CT, and 2 open pilots) found significant improvements in PTSD, anxiety, and depression among survivors of partner abuse, mass disasters, and military service.[33–37]

Mass disasters

Nonprofit organizations have provided yoga programs in disaster areas for decades. Problems of safety and access may account for the paucity of mind-body studies. Nevertheless, a small number of studies demonstrate feasibility, efficacy, and safety of low-cost mind-body treatments for populations affected by mass disasters. In a nonrandomized controlled study, 183 refugees of the 2004 Asian tsunami were assigned by camps to 3 groups:

1. Eight-hour yoga-breath (Breath Water Sound [BWS])
2. BWS plus 3 to 8 hours an exposure therapy called Traumatic Incident Reduction (TIR)
3. Six-week wait list

After 6 weeks, BWS alone and BWS plus TIR reduced the Posttraumatic Stress Disorder Check List-17 (PCL-17) scores by more than 60% and the Beck Depression Index (BDI) more than 90% compared with no change in the control. Most improvements occurred within the first week, with further gains by the 24-week follow-up.[33] Trauma-sensitive programs have been readily accepted by diverse cultures.[35]

Military service related trauma

Among military personnel and veterans, mind-body practices can relieve symptoms of stress, depression, and PTSD. In a rater-blind RCT of 30 Australian Vietnam veterans on disability caused by chronic PTSD, those given a 5-day SKY course had significant reductions on the Clinician Administered PTSD Scale (CAPS) compared with the wait-list control at week 6 and additional substantive improvement at 24 weeks.[37]

Insomnia

Pharmacotherapy for insomnia in geriatric populations entails risks of confusion, cognitive impairment, syncope, and fractures. Mind-body techniques improve sleep safely as show in one RCT.[38] Controlled studies with objective sleep measures are needed.

Depression

A review of yoga for depression reported positive findings in 5 RCTs and advised an optimistic but cautious interpretation.[39] Depression studies with major yoga breathing components include 3 RCTs and 2 open pilots.[40–44] Yoga improved mood in people suffering from clinical depression and increased mental and physical energy, alertness, enthusiasm, and positive mood in healthy individuals.

Obsessive-Compulsive Disorder

ANB usually has a calming effect within 10 minutes. In one RCT and one open trial, patients with obsessive-compulsive disorder (OCD) who were taught Kundalini yoga

Table 1
Breathing practice effects on anxiety, PTSD, OCD, and depression

Study	Design	Subjects	Method: Interventions/Controls	Length	Outcome
STRESS RESPONSE					
Sakakibara and Hayano,[21] 1996	RCT	30 Healthy college students	Audio paced breathing before electric shock INT 1: rate 8 bpm INT 2: 15 bpm CON: nonpaced	5 min	INT 1 ↑ HF-HRV INT 2 ↓ HRV CON ↓ HRV
Malathi and Damodaran,[22] 1999	RCT	50 Medical students examination stress aged 18–19 y	INT 1: yoga postures, breathing, prayer, visualization, meditation INT 2: reading Tested on examination day	3 mo	Yoga group ↓ STAI (*P*<.001)
Nolan et al,[23] 2005	RCT	46 CHD after MI or abnormal stress test	INT 1: paced breathing at 6 bpm with HRV feedback INT 2: relaxation response, autogenic, CBT	5 Sessions 1.5 h each	Similar improvement INT 1 & INT 2 PSS & CES-D
Granath et al,[18] 2006	RCT	40 Swedish employees	INT 1: Kundalini: postures, breathing, prayer INT 2: CBT	4 mo	INT 1 & 2 Similar ↓ in stress, anger, exhaustion, QOL
Gerbarg et al,[24] 2012	Open	84 Health care providers Mississippi after oil spill	BBM training: qigong, coherent breath, resistance breath, breath moving	3 d 18 h	Test d 3 & wk 6 ↓ PSS, EIFI MABI, no change
Afonso et al,[74] 2012	RCT	61 Postmenopausal women with insomnia aged 50–65 y 44 completed	2 sessions per wk 1 h per session INT 1: yoga stretches + fast breathing, relaxation INT 2: passive stretching CON: wait list	Tested at 4 mo	INT 1 greatest ↓ Insomnia, anxiety, depression, QOL, climacteric symptoms

ANXIETY, INSOMNIA

Study	Design	Population	Intervention	Duration	Results
Sahasi et al,[28] 1989	nrCT	91 Anxiety neurosis	INT 1: yoga postures, breath, rest 40 min qd; INT 2: diazepam	3 mo	↓ IPAT greater with yoga (*P*<.05)
Sharma et al,[29] 1991	RCT	71 Anxiety neurosis	INT: yoga; CON: placebo capsule	1 wk Training + daily practice	↓ HAM-A greater with yoga
Manjunath and Telles,[38] 2005	RCT	69 Elderly (aged >60 y) Insomnia	INT1: yoga multi-component; INT2: Ayurvedic herbs; CON: wait list	6 wk	INT1 ↑ 60 min sleep time *P*<.05; INT2 & CON no change
Kuttner et al, 2006	RCT	28 (8 boys/12 girls) adolescents (aged 11–18 y) with IBS	INT: yoga 17 postures + deep breathing; CON: wait list	1 hr Training + 4 wk daily home practice with video	INT trend toward ↓pain ↓GI symptoms, avoidance, RCMAS, FDI, PCQ, CDISF
Telles et al,[30] 2007	Pilot	47 Andaman Island survivors of 2004 tsunami	Ashtanga postures, breathing, meditation	1 wk	↓ fear, anxiety, sadness, insomnia *P*<.05
Kozasa et al,[27] 2008	CT Open	22 Adults c/o anxiety but with no psychiatric diagnoses	INT: Siddha Samadhi yoga: 11 breathing practices 4/2/5/2 n = 14; CON: wait list n = 8	1 mo 40 min per d	INT ↓STAI ↓BDI ↓tension ↑well-being
Telles et al,[31] 2010	RCT	22 Bihar flood survivors with PTSD	INT: like Ashtanga but with more breath practice; CON: wait	1 h per d for 1 wk	INT ↓ sadness; CON: ↑ anxiety
Katzman et al,[25,26] 2012	Pilot Open	31 Adults severe treatment-resistant GAD ± comorbidities	INT: SKY 6 d training + 20 min daily home practice	Tests 6 wk and 6 mo	↓ HAM-A, ↓ ASI, ↓BAI PSWQ↓ all *P*<.001
Katzman et al,[26] 2011	Pilot Open	20 Adults severe treatment-resistant GAD ± comorbidities	BBM 12 h 2 d training + group F/U sessions 60 min twice a month + daily home practice 20 min	Tests 6 wk and 6 mo	↓ BAI, ASI, BDI all *P*<.001; PSWQ *P*<.01

(continued on next page)

Table 1
(continued)

Study	Design	Subjects	Method: Interventions/Controls	Length	Outcome
POST-TRAUMATIC STRESS DISORDER					
Descilo et al,[33] 2010	nrCT	183 Survivors of 2004 SE Asia tsunami with PTSD	INT 1: BWS + SK INT 2: BWS + SK + TIR CON: 6 wk wait list	8 h Tests at 1, 6, 12, and 24 wk	INT 1 & 2 ↓ PCL17 $P<.001$ ↓ BDI $P<.001$ CON: no change
Franzblau et al,[34] 2006	RCT	40 Women abused by intimate partner	INT 1: testimony INT 2: yoga breathing INT 3: testimony + breathing CON: wait list	2 Sessions 45 min/session	FSES 20 INT 3 greatest ↑ Self-efficacy
Gordon et al,[36] 2008	RCT	82 Adolescents with PTSD in postwar Kosovo	Slow breathing, meditation, biofeedback, movement, guided imagery, autogenic training, shaking, drawing, dancing, writing	12 sessions	Intervention group: ↓ PTSD HTQ scores $P<.001$
Carter et al,[37] 2010	RCT	Veterans disabled with chronic PTSD	INT: Sudarshan Kriya CON: 6 wk wait list	5 d	INT: ↓ CAPS Wk 6 $P = .007$ Wk 24 further ↓ CAPS CON: no change
Gerbarg et al,[35] 2011	Pilot Open	17 Adults with depression, anxiety, PTSD related to 2001 WTC attacks	INT: BBM	2 d	↓ BAI, BDI, ASI, all $P<.001$ ↓ PSQI $P<.006$ ↓ SDISL $P<.004$
Gerbarg et al,[35] 2011	Pilot Open	27 Adults[a] 8 y after 2001 WTC attacks GAD, panic, agoraphobia, depression, PTSD	INT: BBM	2 d	↓ BAI ↓ ASI ↓ BDI all $P<.001$

OBSESSIVE COMPULSIVE DISORDER

Study	Type	Sample	Intervention	Duration	Results
Shannahoff-Khalsa et al,[75] 1999	RCT	21 Patients with OCD	INT 1: Kundalini yoga + mantra meditation; INT: relaxation, mindfulness meditation	3 mo, N = 14	INT 1 ↓ Y-BOCS; INT 2 no change
Shannahoff-Khalsa,[45] 2003	Open	11 Patients with OCD	Add: 12 mo Kundalini yoga	15 mo, N = 11	↓ Y-BOCS
DEPRESSION					
Lavey et al,[41] 2005	Open	113 In-patients with MDD, BP, dysthymia, psychosis, borderline	INT: Hatha yoga 45 min once a week for length of hospital stay (average 10 d)	Tested after yoga class	POMS ↓ 5 negative emotions
Janakiramiah et al,[76] 1998	Open	46 Adults with dysthymia	INT: SKY	3 mo	Subjects who practice ≥3 times per wk remitted
Janakiramaiah et al,[44] 2000	RCT	45 Severely depressed hospitalized adults	INT 1: SKY 1 wk training + practice average 5 d per wk; INT 2: imipramine 150 mg/d; INT 3: unipolar ECT 3 times per wk	1 mo	↓ BDI, HAMD; No significant differences between INT 1, INT 2, or INT 3
Tsang et al,[42] 2006	SBRCT	82 Depressed patients aged <65 y	INT 1: relaxation + rhythmic breathing 3 sessions per wk of 30–45 min; CON: newspaper discussion	3 mo	INT 1 ↑ GHQ-12 ↑ Well-being; ↓ Depression; ↑ Self-efficacy

Abbreviations: ASI, Anxiety Sensitivity Index; BAI, Beck Anxiety Inventory; BBM, Breath-Body-Mind workshop; BDI, Beck Depression Inventory; BP, Bipolar; bpm, breaths per minute; BWS, Breath Water Sound; CAPS, Clinician Administered PTSD Scale; CBT, cognitive behavioral therapy; CDISF, Children's Depression Inventory-Short Form; CES-D, Center for Epidemiological Studies Depression Scale; CHD, congestive heart failure; c/o, complain of; CON, control group; ECT, electroconvulsive therapy; EIFI, Exercise Induced Feeling Inventory; FDI, functional disability; FSES, Franzblau Self-Efficacy Scale; F/U, follow-up; GAD, generalized anxiety disorder; GHQ, General health Questionnaire; GI, gastrointestinal; HAM-A, Hamilton Anxiety Rating scale; HAMD, Hamilton Depression Scale; HF-HRV, high-frequency heart rate variability; HRSD, Hamilton Depression Rating Scale; HRV, heart rate variability; HTQ, Harvard Trauma Questionnaire; IBS, Irritable Bowel Syndrome; INT, intervention; IPAT, Institute for Personality and Ability Testing; Anxiety Scale; MABI, Maslach Burnout Inventory; MDD, Major Depressive Disorder; MI, myocardial infarction; nrCT, nonrandomized controlled trial; OCD, obsessive-compulsive disorder; PCQ, Pain Coping Questionnaire; PCL17, Posttraumatic Stress Disorder Check List-17; PCQ, Pain Coping Questionnaire; POMS, Profile of Mood Scale; PSQI, Pittsburg Sleep Quality Index; PSWQ, Penn State Worry Questionnaire; PSS, Perceived Stress Scale; QOL, quality of life; RCMAS, Revised Child Manifest Anxiety Scale; SB, single blinded; SDISL, Sheehan Disability Index Social Life; SK, Sudarshan Kriya; STAI, State-Trait Anxiety Inventory; TIR, trauma incident reduction; WTC, World Trade Center; Y-BOCS, Yale-Brown Obsessive-Compulsive Scale.
[a] First responders, Ground Zero workers, health care providers, tower escapees, witnesses. Mini-mental status examination (MMSE) diagnoses: 14, generalized anxiety disorder; 6, panic; 9, agoraphobia; 12, depression; 23, PTSD.

(slow left-nostril breathing, meditation, and postures) improved significantly on the Yale-Brown Obsessive-Compulsive Scale compared with controls given relaxation and mindfulness meditation.[45] Although left nostril breathing and ANB may be promising adjunctive treatments for anxiety, efficacy in OCD requires 2 to 3 hours of daily practice.

CLINICAL CONSIDERATIONS, RISKS, AND RECOMMENDATIONS
Risks and Contraindications

Among the research studies reviewed here, no adverse reactions to mind-body practices were reported. In general, slow, gentle breath practices are safe in all psychiatric populations. Most patients with asthma are able to benefit from yoga breathing if they are not having acute symptoms. However, at the beginning of slow breathing, such as coherent breathing at 4.5 to 6.5 breaths per minute, in patients with unstable asthma, airways may tend to narrow, exacerbating respiratory problems. One author, Dr Brown, discovered that breath moving (see earlier discussion) keeps airways open during slow breath practices, even in patients with asthma.[46] In patients with chronic obstructive pulmonary disease, rapid breathing can lead to air trapping with increased carbon dioxide (CO_2) levels.

Rapid or forceful breath practices can trigger panic attacks in anxiety disorders, manic episodes in bipolar disorder, flashbacks in PTSD, and altered states of consciousness or psychotic episodes in individuals with a tenuous sense of reality, such as those with schizophrenia, borderline personality disorder, or bipolar disorder. Rapid breath practices may be unsafe during pregnancy and in patients with cardiovascular disease, high blood pressure, lung disease, asthma, seizure disorder, hernia, recent surgery, or recent myocardial infarction.[47]

Hyperventilation, breathing faster or deeper than necessary, lowers serum concentration of CO_2. Novices learning breathing practices tend to exhale too forcefully, particularly during rapid breathing, causing *hypocapnia*, a decline in P_{CO_2}, which can lead to tingling or spasms of the hands and feet, hyperarousal, or altered mental states. Patients with anxiety disorders, acute stress disorder, panic disorder, PTSD, or bipolar disorder tend toward high SNS activity, low PNS activity, low baseline P_{CO_2}, and greater reactivity to changes in P_{CO_2}. Rapid breathing, such as kapalabhati and bhastrika (bellows breath), can increase the risk of panic attacks, flashbacks, or manic states.[48–50] Rapid yoga breathing can increase excretion of lithium causing a drop in serum levels. Patients who are bipolar should avoid rapid yoga breathing.

Reducing the Risks

To minimize the risks of adverse reactions, the following steps are recommended:

1. Assess patients for flashbacks, dissociative episodes, and capacity to maintain the sense of reality. If dissociative episodes are prolonged or involve uncontrolled switching, as in dissociative identity disorder, rapid breathing is contraindicated.
2. If there is a risk of self-injury, psychotherapy and pharmacotherapy can be augmented with calming practices, such as coherent breathing, resistance breathing, or ANB.[20]
3. During slow breath practices, memories or re-experiencing usually are not retraumatizing and can facilitate trauma resolution. Discussing whatever patients experience is helpful.
4. Patients with autonomic instability or over-reactivity, such as war veterans, may need up to 3 months of coherent breathing 20 minutes twice a day and up to 20 minutes of ANB per day to reduce the risk of overwhelming reactions before undertaking more advanced practices.

Mind-Body Techniques in Clinical Practice

Clinician preparation

Clinicians who learn basic breath practices before introducing them into treatment are better equipped to counsel patients regarding the choice of techniques and maintaining compliance. Patients who cannot access a trainer may start with books and CDs. However, the authors find teaching patients within therapy sessions more effective than letting them learn it on their own.

Begin with simple, safe, effective breath practices

Coherent breathing is a simple effective introductory practice. Patients can purchase a CD, such as Respire-1 (Coherence LLC, Pilot Point, Texas; www.coherence.com), or a breath pacer (see "Technology-assisted breathing interventions"), follow the paced breathing at 4.5 to 6.5 breaths per minute (bpm), and experience gentle relaxation with no adverse effects. Prescribe 10 or 20 minutes twice a day plus additional practice as needed.

TECHNOLOGY-ASSISTED BREATHING INTERVENTIONS

Nowhere has the merger of Eastern and Western practices been more apparent than in the surge of technology-based programs and devices to facilitate therapeutic breathing practices. These programs and devices include guided audio or video tutorials, Web-based and mobile customizable breathing pacers, computer-based and mobile physiologic monitoring, and feedback systems. This review focuses on technology-assisted interventions that primarily support breath training with minimal instruction in other modalities.

Background, Physiology, Systems, and Definitions

Numerous studies indicate that most people can accurately follow paced breathing instructions with brief training[12,51] and that paced breathing using audio and video cues can produce acute physiologic improvements and reductions in symptoms of arousal and anxiety.[13,52,53] There are nearly 100 breath pacing applications for mobile phones; but to the authors' knowledge, there are no clinical trials examining their effects on psychiatric conditions. The main drawback of these unassisted breath pacing tools is that without clinician support, there is no feedback to guide individuals who may need assistance in performing the breathing practices correctly. In contrast, breath-retraining biofeedback systems offer individualized feedback using targeted physiologic parameters (eg, respiration rate, HRV, and end-tidal CO_2), which are either directly related to respiration or highly correlated with changes in respiration.

Biofeedback protocols often include a respiratory strain gauge (pneumograph) because it provides direct assessment of the respiratory rate rather than relying on a correlated variable, such as HRV or skin temperature. This gauge obviates confounding factors, such as thoracic breathing (breathing into the upper chest without expanding the lower part of the lungs) or reverse breathing (contracting the abdomen during inhalation instead of during exhalation).[52] Although many studies treating mental health problems include a respiratory strain gauge as a training tool, the majority using it as a stand-alone device targeting cardiovascular disease.[52] HRV biofeedback and respiratory feedback with capnometry (measurement of exhaled end tidal CO_2 levels using a nasal canula) also use breath retraining as the primary modality. HRV, based on the rate of change of the heart's interbeat interval, is used as a primary indicator of cardiovascular health. HRV biofeedback is typically performed by sampling the real-time heart rate and displaying its natural increases during inspiration and decreases during expiration (a phenomenon called respiratory sinus arrhythmia) on the screen along with a Fourier transformation of the HRV data into frequency spectrums. HRV biofeedback aims to reduce breathing frequency to a rate unique to the individual such that real-time heart rate and respiration covary in a perfect phase relationship, creating a sine wave heart rate pattern and a unimodal spike in low-frequency HRV at 0.1 Hz, indicating maximal HRV and sympathovagal balance.[54,55] This unique breathing rate between 4.5 to 6.5 bpm is called *resonance frequency*.[54] Although studies using these types of devices for medical disorders have been more rigorous, small, randomized pilots report benefits in a range of psychiatric disorders (**Table 2**).

Anxiety, Stress, Performance, Panic Disorder, PTSD, and Depression

Anxiety, stress, performance

Small pilot studies found that HRV biofeedback and respiratory strain gauge biofeedback can induce immediate reductions in anxiety and arousal similar to guided breath training without devices. In 2 single-blind studies, control group participants were instructed to use a concentrative mindfulness device while letting go of stressful thoughts. All groups in both studies significantly reduced state anxiety and stress levels, but changes were significantly greater in the HRV intervention compared with the control. Moreover, the more efficient individuals were at mastering the breathing technique, the greater the reductions in state anxiety.[56,57] Although breath retraining reduces overall arousal and anxiety, cognitive techniques or other strategies may also be needed, depending on the capacities of the individual.[58] Some studies in normal populations suggest that short-term breathing-based biofeedback may yield longer-term improvements in stress, performance anxiety, and cognitive functioning; but more evidence is needed to validate the purported physiologic mechanisms of long-term change.[59] In 2 studies, respiratory strain gauge biofeedback or HRV biofeedback improved the quality of life for patients with cardiovascular disease compared with control.[60,61]

Panic disorder

Several small studies and one RCT used capnometer and strain gauge feedback to reduce panic attacks and hyperventilation. During shallow rapid breathing, hyperventilation (see earlier discussion) can lead to hypocapnia and pH imbalance (increased blood alkalinity) with blood vessel constriction, reducing brain oxygen levels. Capnometry is a prime assessment and intervention tool because rapid breathing creates low end-tidal CO_2, whereas slow therapeutic breathing normalizes the gas exchange. Slow breathing and capnometry-assisted breathing relieve hypocapnia.[62] In an RCT, capnometry-assisted respiratory training was equivalent to cognitive therapy in reducing panic symptoms. However, capnometry-assisted training, but not cognitive training, normalized hypocapnia, suggesting that breath retraining is a useful adjunct to cognitive treatments in panic disorder.[63]

PTSD

Individuals with PTSD have a low baseline HRV.[64] In a 4-week RCT of 38 patients with PTSD, the HRV biofeedback group had significantly greater improvements in resting HRV and depressive symptoms compared with a progressive muscle relaxation group.[65] In another RCT, HRV augmentation of a trauma reduction program (TRP) reduced PTSD scores and avoidance/numbing significantly more than TRP alone. Increased HRV was associated with reduced PTSD scores.[66]

Depression

Two small single group studies and one RCT found device-guided HRV feedback beneficial for depression. In a 2-month RCT, HRV feedback significantly reduced depressive symptoms versus progressive muscle relaxation.[67] In an open trial, HRV biofeedback significantly improved fibromyalgia and depression at the 3-month follow-up, showing potential longer-term benefits.[68]

CLINICAL CONSIDERATIONS

Advantages of Technology-Assisted Breath Retraining Devices

Studies are building an evidence base for the benefits of technology-assisted therapeutic breathing as a stand-alone and/or adjunctive treatment of psychiatric disorders. Technology-assisted breathing devices open the world of therapeutic breathing to individuals who might not pursue traditional guided practices, such as yoga. For example, Muench[69] reported that men are more likely than women to prefer a portable biofeedback device to other relaxation practices. Perhaps the tangible, gadgetlike quality is more appealing to men. Also, many find it easier to stay on task with technology-assisted practices versus unguided breathing or meditation. Another advantage of device-guided applications is inclusion of a history of use that facilitates honest communication about barriers to practice, increases accountability, and enhances compliance with homework. With the increase of continuous passive monitoring devices, individuals will soon be able to receive notifications to practice therapeutic breathing when changes occur in their physiology.[70–72]

Limitations, Precautions, and Contraindications

Untested breathing applications using features embedded in mobile phones are flooding the market. Innovative mobile phone applications include detecting respiratory rates as the user breathes into the microphone, using the accelerometer to detect respiratory rates by placing the phone on one's abdomen, and using the camera as a real-time HR sensor to display HRV. These options are intriguing, but their reliability is questionable until validated with standard monitoring equipment.

Patient factors

Approximately 10% of people experience biofeedback-induced anxiety while attempting (usually unsuccessfully) to alter their physiology through breathing.[57,73] Because many factors affect physiology (eg, blood pressure–regulating medications) and some individuals are prone to dyspnea, certain assistive technologies may not be suitable or may require additional in-person instruction.

Patient and clinician factors: cost and accessibility, ease of use

The cost of breath training programs and devices ranges from $100 to $2000 or more, with considerable differences in their capabilities. Patients can purchase portable devices from $100 to $300 that offer real-time feedback (usually on a single physiologic variable) or choose simple breath retraining phone applications that may or may not provide feedback. It is important for clinicians to evaluate risks and benefits for each patient and to learn how to use devices properly before recommending them. Patients are far more likely to benefit when given some personal instruction and monitoring by their health care provider. For information on breath retraining devices, protocols, and referrals, one can visit the Web sites of the Association for Applied Psychophysiology and Biofeedback and the Quantified Self Guide to Self-Tracking Tools.

Table 2
Clinical studies of technology-assisted breathing devices in psychiatric disorders

Study	Design	Subjects	Method: Intervention/Controls	Length	Outcome[a]
Anxiety/Stress (Ib efficiacy)					
Morarend et al,[58] 2011	RCT	81 Patients with dental anxiety	INT: respiratory strain gauge device (ambulatory) CON: no treatment	15 min	INT: ↓ VAS negative feelings about dental injection; no change CSAS, DISS CON: no change
Sherlin et al,[56,57] 2009, 2010	RCT (SB)	43 Individuals with high levels of perceived stress	INT 1: HRV biofeedback device (ambulatory) ACON: passive concentrative control device (ambulatory)	15 min	INT 1 >ACON: ↓ STAI-S, ↓ HR & ↑ alpha waves in anterior cingulated cortex
Sutarto et al, 2010	Pilot study	9 Female university students	INT: 6 sessions of HRV biofeedback (office based + home practice) ACON: no treatment	3 wk	INT: ↑ verbal memory & mathematical decision making CON: no changes
Prinsaloo et al, 2011	RCT (SB)	18 Individuals reporting high perceived stress	INT 1: HRV biofeedback device (ambulatory) ACON: passive concentrative device (ambulatory)	15 min	INT >ACON: ↑ subjective feelings of relaxation (SRI); ↑ scores cognitive task (MST) INT 1 & ACON: ↓ STAI-S; ↑ SRI
Lemaire et al, 2011	RCT	40 Physicians	INT: social support + HRV biofeedback CON: social support visits only	28 d	INT >CON: ↓ global perceptions of work-related stress
Ratanasiripong et al, 2012	RCT	60 Nursing students	INT: HRV biofeedback device (ambulatory) CON: no treatment	5 wk	INT: ↓ STAI-S & PSS CON: no changes
Meuret et al,[63] 2009, 2010	RCT	41 Patients with panic disorder	INT 1: capnometry-assisted respiratory training INT 2: cognitive therapy	5 wk	INT 1 & INT 2: ↓PDSS; ↓ACQ; ↓STAI INT 1 >INT 2: ↓ hypocapnic breathing

PTSD (IIa efficacy)

Study	Type	Sample	Intervention	Duration	Outcomes
Zucker et al,[65] 2009	RCT	38 Individuals in drug treatment with elevated PTSD scores	INT 1: HRV biofeedback device (ambulatory); INT 2: progressive muscle relaxation audio training	4 wk	INT 1 >INT 2: ↓ BDI; ↑ HRV; INT 1 & INT 2: ↓ PCL; ↓ ISI
Tan et al, 2010	RCT	20 Veterans with PTSD	INT 1: TRP + 8 office-based HRV biofeedback sessions + home practice; TAU CON: TRP only	8 wk	INT >CON: ↓ PCL avoidance & numbing subscale; INT 1 & TAU CON: ↓ PCL

Depression (Ib efficacy)

Study	Type	Sample	Intervention	Duration	Outcomes
Karavidas et al, 2007	Pilot study	11 Individuals with MDD	Single pilot group: office-based HRV biofeedback + home practice	10 sessions	INT ↓ BDI & HAM-D; ↑ HRV
Seipmann et al, 2008	Pilot study	14 Patients with varying degrees of depression; 12 Healthy adults	6 Office-based HRV biofeedback sessions + home practice	2 wk	Depressed group: ↓ BDI; ↓ STAI; ↑ HRV; Healthy group: no changes
Rene,[67] 2008	RCT	32 Women enrolled in welfare-to-work program	INT 1: HRV biofeedback device (ambulatory); INT 2: daily progressive muscle relaxation audio training	8 wk	INT 1 >INT 2: ↓ BDI; ↑ employment and motivation; INT 1 & INT 2: ↓ ISI
Hasset et al,[68] 2007	Pilot study	12 Women with fibromyalgia	10 Weekly sessions of HRV Biofeedback	12 wk	INT ↓ BDI & MPQ; ↑ overall functioning

Abbreviations: ACON, active control group; ACQ, Anxiety Control Questionnaire; ASI, Anxiety Sensitivity Index; BAI, Beck Anxiety inventory; CDAS, Corah Dental Anxiety Scale; CON, control group; DISS, Dental Injection Sensitivity Survey (Krochak and Friedman, 1998); HAM-D+, Hamilton Depression Rating scale; HRV: heart rate variability; INT: intervention; INT 1: main Intervention; INT 2: Alternate Intervention; INT 1 > INT 2, significantly greater change in INT 1 compared with INT 2; INT 1 & INT 2: significant changes within groups but not between groups ambulatory: device used at home; IIa efficacy: evidence from at least one well-performed study with control group; Ib efficacy: evidence from at least one randomized study with control; MPQ: McGill Pain Questionnaire; PDSS: Panic Disorder Sensitivity Scale; SB, single blinded; SRI, Smith Relaxation Inventory; STAI: State-Trait Anxiety Inventory; TAU: treatment as usual; TRP, trauma reduction program; UP, unpublished; VAS: visual analog scale.

[a] NOTE: All findings presented are statistically significant.

SUMMARY

The empiric literature on therapeutic breathing for psychiatric disorders is expanding along with the breath retraining technologies. Clinicians interested in integrating breath practices into their work will be able to choose applications that they find most suitable to their patient population and to their own practice style. As with other treatment decisions, the choice of technology should take into consideration the evidence of efficacy, reliability, cost, ease of use, interests of the clinician, patient preferences, patient motivation, risk factors, and capacities to learn these new techniques.

APPENDIX: REFERENCES

Supplemental References 74–76 are available at http://www.psych.theclinics.com/dx. doi.org/10.1016/j.psc.2013.01.001.

REFERENCES

1. Telles S, Desiraju T. Heart rate alterations in different types of pranayamas. Indian J Physiol Pharmacol 1992;36(4):287–8.
2. Telles S, Nagarathna R, Nagendra HR, et al. Physiological changes in sports teachers following 3 months of training in yoga. Indian J Med Sci 1993;47(10): 235–8.
3. Uebelacker LA, Epstein-Lubow G, Gaudiano BA, et al. Hatha yoga for depression: critical review of the evidence for efficacy, plausible mechanisms of action, and directions for future research. J Psychiatr Pract 2010;16(1):22–33.
4. Vasiliev V. Let every breath. Secrets of the Russian breath masters. Richmond Hill (Ontario): Russian Martial Art; 2006.
5. Hanh TN. You are here. Discovering the magic of the present moment. 1st edition. Boston, London: ShambhalaPublications, Inc; 2009.
6. Brown RP, Gerbarg PL. Sudarshan Kriya yogic breathing in the treatment of stress, anxiety, and depression: part I-neurophysiologic model. J Altern Complement Med 2005;11(1):189–201.
7. Brown RP, Gerbarg PL. Sudarshan Kriya yogic breathing in the treatment of stress, anxiety, and depression. Part II–clinical applications and guidelines. J Altern Complement Med 2005;11(4):711–7.
8. Streeter CC, Gerbarg PL, Saper RB, et al. Effects of yoga on the autonomic nervous system, gamma-aminobutyric-acid, and allostasis in epilepsy, depression, and post-traumatic stress disorder. Med Hypotheses 2012;78(5):571–9.
9. Brown RP, Gerbarg PL. Yoga breathing, meditation, and longevity. Ann N Y Acad Sci 2009;1172:54–62.
10. Bernardi L, Porta C, Gabutti A, et al. Modulatory effects of respiration. Auton Neurosci 2001;90(1–2):47–56.
11. Lehrer P, Karavidas MK, Lu SE, et al. Voluntarily produced increases in heart rate variability modulate autonomic effects of endotoxin induced systemic inflammation: an exploratory study. Appl Psychophysiol Biofeedback 2010;35(4):303–15.
12. Song HS, Lehrer PM. The effects of specific respiratory rates on heart rate and heart rate variability. Appl Psychophysiol Biofeedback 2003;28(1):13–23.
13. Vaschillo EG, Vaschillo B, Lehrer PM. Characteristics of resonance in heart rate variability stimulated by biofeedback. Appl Psychophysiol Biofeedback 2006; 31(2):129–42.
14. Telles S, Nagarathna R, Nagendra HR. Autonomic changes during "OM" meditation. Indian J Physiol Pharmacol 1995;39(4):418–20.

15. Kalyani BG, Venkatasubramanian G, Arasappa R, et al. Neurohemodynamic correlates of 'OM' chanting: a pilot functional magnetic resonance imaging study. Int J Yoga 2011;4(1):3–6.
16. Craig AD. Interoception: the sense of the physiological condition of the body. Curr Opin Neurobiol 2003;13(4):500–5.
17. Hopper JW, Frewen PA, van der Kolk BA, et al. Neural correlates of reexperiencing, avoidance, and dissociation in PTSD: symptom dimensions and emotion dysregulation in responses to script-driven trauma imagery. J Trauma Stress 2007;20(5):713–25.
18. Granath J, Ingvarsson S, von Thiele U, et al. Stress management: a randomized study of cognitive behavioural therapy and yoga. Cogn Behav Ther 2006;35(1):3–10.
19. Michalsen A, Grossman P, Acil A, et al. Rapid stress reduction and anxiolysis among distressed women as a consequence of a three-month intensive yoga program. Med Sci Monit 2005;11(12):CR555–61.
20. Gerbarg PL. Yoga and neuro-psychoanalysis. In: Anderson FS, editor. Bodies in treatment: the unspoken dimension. Hillsdale (NJ): The Analytic Press, Inc; 2008. p. 127–50.
21. Sakakibara M, Hayano J. Effect of slowed respiration on cardiac parasympathetic response to threat. Psychosom Med 1996;58(1):32–7.
22. Malathi A, Damodaran A. Stress due to exams in medical students–role of yoga. Indian J Physiol Pharmacol 1999;43(2):218–24.
23. Nolan RP, Kamath MV, Floras JS, et al. Heart rate variability biofeedback as a behavioral neurocardiac intervention to enhance vagal heart rate control. Am Heart J 2005;149(6):1137.
24. Gerbarg PL, Streeter CC, Whitfield T, et al. Breath-body-mind (B-B-M) training for healthcare providers post 2010 Gulf oil spill. 16th Annual Meeting American Psychiatric Association. Philadelphia, May 5–9, 2012.
25. Katzman MA, Vermani M, Gerbarg PL, et al. A multicomponent yoga-based, breath intervention program as an adjunctive treatment in patients suffering from Generalized Anxiety Disorder (GAD) with or without comorbidities. Int J Yoga 2012;5(1):57–65.
26. Katzman MA, Vermani M, Gerbarg PL, et al. Breath-Body-Mind workshop as adjunctive treatment in patients suffering from Generalized Anxiety Disorder (GAD) with or without comorbidities. Presented at the American Psychiatric Association Annual Meeting. Honolulu, Hawaii, May 14–18, 2011.
27. Kozasa EH, Santos RF, Rueda AD, et al. Evaluation of Siddha Samadhi yoga for anxiety and depression symptoms: a preliminary study. Psychol Rep 2008;103(1):271–4.
28. Sahasi G, Moha D, Kacker C. Effectiveness of yogic techniques in the management of anxiety. J Pers Clin Stud 1989;5:51–5.
29. Sharma I, Azmi SA, Settiwar RM. Evaluation of the effect of pranayama in anxiety states. Alternative Med 1991;3:227–35.
30. Telles S, Naveen KV, Dash M. Yoga reduces symptoms of distress in tsunami survivors in the Andaman islands. Evid Based Complement Alternat Med 2007;4(4):503–9.
31. Telles S, Singh N, Joshi M, et al. Post traumatic stress symptoms and heart rate variability in Bihar flood survivors following yoga: a randomized controlled study. BMC Psychiatry 2010;10:18.
32. Fehmi LR, Robbins J. The open focus brain. harnessing the power of attention to heal mind and body. Westminster (MD): Random House, Inc; 2008.

33. Descilo T, Vedamurtachar A, Gerbarg PL, et al. Effects of a yoga breath intervention alone and in combination with an exposure therapy for post-traumatic stress disorder and depression in survivors of the 2004 South-East Asia tsunami. Acta Psychiatr Scand 2010;121(4):289–300.

34. Franzblau SH, Smith M, Echevarria S, et al. Take a breath, break the silence: the effects of yogic breathing and testimony about battering on feelings of self-efficacy in battered women. Int J Yoga Therap 2006;16:49–57.

35. Gerbarg PL, Wallace G, Brown RP. Mass disasters and mind-body solutions: evidence and field insights. Int J Yoga Therap 2011;(21):97–107.

36. Gordon JS, Staples JK, Blyta JK, et al. Treatment of post-traumatic stress disorder in postwar Kosovo adolescents using mind-body skills groups: a randomized controlled study. J Clin Psychiatry 2008;9:1469–76.

37. Carter JJ, Gerbarg PL, Brown RP, et al. Multi-component yoga breath based program reduces PTSD in Vietnam War veterans. Annual Meeting American Psychiatric Association. New Orleans, May 22–26, 2010.

38. Manjunath NK, Telles S. Influence of yoga and Ayurveda on self-rated sleep in a geriatric population. Indian J Med Res 2005;121(5):683–90.

39. Pilkington K, Kirkwood G, Rampes H, et al. Yoga for depression: the research evidence. J Affect Disord 2005;89(1–3):13–24.

40. Khumar SS, Kaur P, Kaur S. Effectiveness of Shavasana on depression among university students. Indian J Clin Psychol 1993;20(2):82–7.

41. Lavey R, Sherman T, Mueser KT, et al. The effects of yoga on mood in psychiatric inpatients. Psychiatr Rehabil J 2005;28(4):399–402.

42. Tsang HW, Fung KM, Chan AS, et al. Effect of a qigong exercise programme on elderly with depression. Int J Geriatr Psychiatry 2006;21(9):890–7.

43. Wood C. Mood change and perceptions of vitality: a comparison of the effects of relaxation, visualization and yoga. J R Soc Med 1993;86(5):254–8.

44. Janakiramaiah N, Gangadhar BN, Naga Venkatesha Murthy PJ, et al. Antidepressant efficacy of Sudarshan Kriya yoga (SKY) in melancholia: a randomized comparison with electroconvulsive therapy (ECT) and imipramine. J Affect Disord 2000;57(1–3):255–9.

45. Shannahoff-Khalsa DS. Kundalini yoga meditation techniques for the treatment of obsessive-compulsive and OC spectrum disorders. Brief Treatment and Crisis Intervention 2003;3:369–82.

46. Brown RP, Gerbarg PL. The healing power of the breath. simple techniques to reduce stress and anxiety, enhance concentration, and balance your emotions. Boston: Shambhala Publications, Inc; 2012.

47. Brown RP, Gerbarg PL, Muskin PR. How to use herbs, nutrients, and yoga in mental health care. New York: W. W. Norton & Company; 2009.

48. Raghuraj P, Ramakrishnan AG, Nagendra HR, et al. Effect of two selected yogic breathing techniques of heart rate variability. Indian J Physiol Pharmacol 1998; 42(4):467–72.

49. Stancak AJ, Kuna M. EEG changes during forced alternate nostril breathing. Int J Psychophysiol 1994;18(1):75–9.

50. Telles S, Raghuraj P, Arankalle D, et al. Immediate effect of high-frequency yoga breathing on attention. Indian J Med Sci 2008;62(1):20–2.

51. Clark ME, Hirschman R. Effects of paced respiration on anxiety reduction in a clinical population. Appl Psychophysiol Biofeedback 1990;15(3):273–84.

52. Gavish B. Device-guided breathing in the home setting: technology, performance and clinical outcomes. Biol Psychol 2010;84(1):150–6.

53. Strauss Blasche G, Moser M, Voica M, et al. Relative timing of inspiration and expiration affects respiratory sinus arrhythmia. Clin Exp Pharmacol Physiol 2001;27(8):601–6.

54. Lehrer PM, Vaschillo E, Vaschillo B. Resonant frequency biofeedback training to increase cardiac variability: rationale and manual for training. Appl Psychophysiol Biofeedback 2000;25(3):177–91.

55. Vaschillo E, Vaschillo B, Lehrer P. Heartbeat synchronizes with respiratory rhythm only under specific circumstances. Chest 2004;126(4):1385–7.

56. Sherlin L, Gevirtz R, Wyckoff S, et al. Effects of respiratory sinus arrhythmia biofeedback versus passive biofeedback control. Int J Stress Manag 2009; 16(3):233.

57. Sherlin L, Muench F, Wyckoff S. Respiratory sinus arrhythmia feedback in a stressed population exposed to a brief stressor demonstrated by quantitative EEG and sLORETA. Appl Psychophysiol Biofeedback 2010;35(3):219–28.

58. Morarend QA, Spector ML, Dawson DV, et al. The use of a respiratory rate biofeedback device to reduce dental anxiety: an exploratory investigation. Appl Psychophysiol Biofeedback 2011;36(2):63–70.

59. Wheat AL, Larkin KT. Biofeedback of heart rate variability and related physiology: a critical review. Appl Psychophysiol Biofeedback 2010;35(3):229–42.

60. Giardino ND, Chan L, Borson S. Combined heart rate variability and pulse oximetry biofeedback for chronic obstructive pulmonary disease: preliminary findings. Appl Psychophysiol Biofeedback 2004;29(2):121–33.

61. Parati G, Malfatto G, Boarin S, et al. Device-guided paced breathing in the home setting: effects on exercise capacity, pulmonary and ventricular function in patients with chronic heart failure: a pilot study. Circ Heart Fail 2008;1(3):178.

62. Grossman P, De Swart J, Defares P. A controlled study of a breathing therapy for treatment of hyperventilation syndrome. J Psychosom Res 1985;29(1):49–58.

63. Meuret AE, Rosenfield D, Seidel A, et al. Respiratory and cognitive mediators of treatment change in panic disorder: evidence for intervention specificity. J Consult Clin Psychol 2010;78(5):691.

64. Gevirtz R, Dalenberg C. Heart rate variability biofeedback in the treatment of trauma symptoms. Biofeedback 2008;36(1):22–3.

65. Zucker TL, Samuelson KW, Muench F, et al. The effects of respiratory sinus arrhythmia biofeedback on heart rate variability and posttraumatic stress disorder symptoms: a pilot study. Appl Psychophysiol Biofeedback 2009;34(2):135–43.

66. Tan G, Dao TK, Farmer L, et al. Heart rate variability (HRV) and posttraumatic stress disorder (PTSD): a pilot study. Appl Psychophysiol Biofeedback 2011; 36(1):27–35.

67. Rene R. HRV Biofeedback vs PMR in reducing depression in low income women. 39th Annual Conference of the Association for Applied Psychophysiology and Biofeedback. Daytona Beach, 2008.

68. Hassett AL, Radvanski DC, Vaschillo EG, et al. A pilot study of the efficacy of heart rate variability (HRV) biofeedback in patients with fibromyalgia. Appl Psychophysiol Biofeedback 2007;32(1):1–10.

69. Muench F. HRV: the manufacturers and vendors speak. 2008.

70. Fletcher RR, Dobson K, Goodwin MS, et al. iCalm: wearable sensor and network architecture for wirelessly communicating and logging autonomic activity. IEEE Trans Inf Technol Biomed 2010;14(2):215–23.

71. AlKhalidi HR, Hong Y, Fleming TR, et al. Insights on the robust variance estimator under recurrent events model. Biometrics 2011;67(4):1564–72.

72. Moraveji N, Olson B, Nguyen T, et al, editors. Peripheral paced respiration: influencing user physiology during information work. Proceedings of the 24th annual ACM Symposium on User Interface Software and Technology. ACM; 2011.

73. Allen B. What resonates with you?: methods of induced cardiovascular resonance. University Libraries, Virginia Polytechnic Institute and State University; 2010.

Mindfulness Meditation Practices as Adjunctive Treatments for Psychiatric Disorders

William R. Marchand, MD

KEYWORDS

• Mindfulness • Meditation • Depression • Anxiety

KEY POINTS

- Mindfulness is nonjudgmental moment-by-moment awareness of sensations, thoughts, and emotions.
- A mindfulness meditation practice may decrease symptoms of depression and anxiety as well as enhance psychological well-being.
- Mindfulness-based stress reduction and mindfulness-based cognitive therapy are evidence-based interventions that can be used as adjunctive interventions for mood and anxiety disorders.

INTRODUCTION

There is an expanding body of literature documenting trials of mindfulness interventions as adjunctive treatments for psychiatric disorders. In particular, mindfulness-based stress reduction (MBSR) and mindfulness-based cognitive therapy (MBCT) have been studied as clinical interventions and have a strong evidence base documenting their effectiveness. This review provides an overview of Buddhist meditation practices, MBSR, and MBCT, and offers recommendations in regard to how clinicians can support patients who are enrolled in a mindfulness course.

OVERVIEW OF MINDFULNESS INTERVENTIONS AND MECHANISMS OF ACTION
Meditation

Meditation has been practiced since ancient times as a component of numerous spiritual traditions. Meditation can refer to a specific practice or a mental state induced as

Funding: This work was supported by a Department of Veterans Affairs Career Development Award. Additional support was provided by the resources and the use of facilities at the VA Salt Lake City Health Care System.
Conflict of Interest: None.
George E. Wahlen Veterans Administration Medical Center, 500 Foothill, Salt Lake City, UT 84148, USA
E-mail address: wmarchand@me.com

Psychiatr Clin N Am 36 (2013) 141–152
http://dx.doi.org/10.1016/j.psc.2013.01.002   **psych.theclinics.com**
0193-953X/13/$ – see front matter Published by Elsevier Inc.

a result of that practice. Today, the word meditation is often used as a general term for a variety of practices generally aimed at focusing attention and awareness to voluntarily control mental processes.[1] These practices may be part of a religious or spiritual tradition or may be secular in nature.

Mindfulness

Mindfulness is style of meditative practice. However, mindfulness more generally means a mental state whereby nonjudgmental awareness is specifically focused on one's moment-by-moment experience.[2] The state of mindfulness may occur during the practice of mindfulness meditation or at any time one intentionally focuses awareness on the present moment. Mindfulness meditation can be thought of as a framework used to develop the state of mindfulness.[3]

Mindfulness is the intentional focusing of one's attention on awareness of the present moment. This awareness encompasses physical sensations of external sensory inputs and interoception (awareness of internal bodily sensations). Furthermore, attention is specifically focused on the internal workings of the mind,[4] including cognitions and emotions. During mindfulness one becomes an observer of one's own stream of consciousness.

MBSR and MBCT

MBSR and MBCT are secular, clinically based group therapy methods using manuals and standardized techniques.

MBSR was developed by Dr Jon Kabat-Zinn at the University of Massachusetts Medical Center.[4] MBSR includes education about stress as well as training on coping strategies and assertiveness. The mindfulness component includes sitting meditation, a body scan, and Hatha Yoga. MBSR involves the cultivation of several attitudes, including becoming an impartial witness to one's own experience and acceptance of things as they actually are in the present moment.[4]

MBCT was developed by Zindel Segal, Mark Williams, and John Teasdale.[5] MBCT is based on MBSR and combines the principles of cognitive therapy with those of mindfulness. It was developed specifically to prevent relapse of depression. MBCT uses secular mindfulness techniques including seated meditation. The program specifically teaches recognition of deteriorating mood with the aim of disengaging from self-perpetuating patterns of ruminative, negative thought that contribute to depressive relapse.[5]

Buddhist Philosophy and Contemplative Practices

MBSR and MBCT are secular interventions with origins in Buddhist spiritual practices.[6] Although all references to spirituality in general and Buddhism in particular have been removed from both, some familiarity with Buddhist philosophy may help explicate the rationale for using these approaches for individuals with a variety of psychiatric symptoms.

According to Buddhist philosophy, humans are inherently dissatisfied and suffer unnecessarily because of a fundamental misperception of reality. This misunderstanding occurs because of the normal human tendency toward an egocentric worldview. In this way of thinking, "egocentric" does not imply selfishness or conceit. It simply means that to survive and prosper, humans have evolved in such a way that there is propensity to view the world in the context of meeting one's own needs. This view supports the survival of both the individual and the species. However, it also fosters a strong sense of, and attachment to, the concept of an independent and separate self. Buddhism posits that the attachment to the concept of an independent and separate self results in a worldview that is inconsistent with lasting happiness or satisfaction.

Attachment to the concept of self is thought to lead to unhappiness in several ways. Foremost of these is impermanence. We will all ultimately die and lose everything that we love in this lifetime. Hence, the strength of attachment to the concept of self tends to be associated with a sense of anxiety associated with the inevitable eventual loss of self through death.

Self-Referential Thinking in Mood and Anxiety Disorders

As reviewed elsewhere,[7] a large body of literature indicates an association between dysfunctional self-referential thinking and both mood and anxiety disorders. For example, aberrant self-schemas form the basis for some models of the psychology of depression. Numerous studies indicate an association between low self-concept and/or negative self-schemas and depression, and suggest that self-referential thinking is abnormal in affective illness.

In addition to negative self-concept, the amount of self-referential thinking seems to be associated with affective symptoms. Excessive self-focus in general is associated with negative affect[8] and unipolar depression is associated with an increase in self-focused thinking.[9,10]

The type of self-referential thinking is also important. Narrative self-reference is a mode of thinking that includes both memories of the past and intentions for the future.[11] The narrative sense of self is composed of memories of subjective experiences linked across time. An important point is that narrative self-reference often occurs as stimulus-independent thought (SIT). SIT is a component of mind wandering[12] and is automatic, and occurs in the absence of a strong requirement to respond to external stimuli.[13] Such stimulus-independent thinking may take the form of self-referential rumination[14–17] and is analytical (thinking analytically about self and symptoms). The narrative/analytical type of self-referential thinking is mostly maladaptive[18] and is frequently associated with generalized autobiographical memory,[19] negative self-judgments,[20] and dysphoria.[21,22] Furthermore, self-focused rumination is specifically associated with depression.[14–17]

Psychological Mechanisms of Mindfulness

Mindfulness practices aim to develop experiential self-reference, which is adaptive.[19,23] In contrast to the analytical/narrative style of self-referential thinking, experiential self-reference is the experience of self in the immediate moment without a storyline. As reviewed elsewhere,[7] mindfulness is associated with decreased rumination, and evidence indicates that benefits of practice are associated with both decreased rumination and increased mindfulness. Thus, mindfulness may lead to enhanced psychological well-being by decreasing rumination in general, and perhaps specifically by decreasing the amount and type of attention focused on the self.

The practice of mindfulness may change self-referential thinking through the psychological mechanism of reperceiving.[24] In a model developed by Shapiro and colleagues,[24] reperceiving is defined as a fundamental shift in perspective. As a result of this shift, one is able to step back from one's own thoughts and emotions. In other words, one becomes an observer of one's own mental processes. During the practice of mindfulness, moment-by-moment nonjudgmental awareness is focused on thoughts and emotions as well as on internal and external physical sensations. By practicing open awareness, one may begin to see the true nature of thoughts as transient phenomena that often have little or no validity. This process extends to the thoughts that arise about the concept of self. Ultimately, practitioners may develop a different relationship with cognitions in general and self-referential thinking in particular. The result is a dis-identification with one's mental processes. Becoming less identified with one's emotions and cognitions results in these mental processes losing power. For example, negative thoughts may be less likely to lead to depression. Moreover, reperceiving may also lead to a realization that self is only a psychological construct made up of changing recollections, attitudes, sensations, and viewpoints.[24] Hence, mindfulness may facilitate less identification with the concept of self and less attachment to an egocentric worldview. Ultimately, one may experience less suffering when the self is threatened, whether the threat is actual or perceived.

Evidence suggests that mindfulness practice is associated with enhanced emotional self-regulation and decreased emotional reactivity.[25–31] Reperceiving allows one to stand back and observe, rather than be controlled by, the unpleasant sensations.[24] This shift in perspective may facilitate the ability to self-regulate by allowing the use of adaptive coping skills and preventing maladaptive responses. Gaining some distance from negative thoughts, emotions, and sensations may enable the use of positive coping strategies rather than simply reacting. In addition, an increased ability to tolerate uncomfortable emotions or sensations may result in greater exposure to the discomfort and, thus, eventual desensitization. Cognitive and behavioral flexibility may also facilitate more adaptive responding in general. Clarification of values may result in choosing behaviors more congruent with one's core values.[24]

Neural Processes Altered by Mindfulness and Meditation

In addition to the psychological mechanisms described, an expanding body of literature now indicates that meditation and mindfulness affect brain function. Some of these findings have been reviewed in detail elsewhere,[7] and a brief summation is provided here.

The amygdala is thought to function as a salience and/or threat detector. Amygdala output results in fear-related behaviors, and is associated with both anxiety and depression. Some evidence indicates that mindfulness practices alter amygdala activation and therefore may decrease emotional reactivity by modulating amygdala output.[7]

Most of the medial cortex has been characterized as an anatomic and functional unit known as the cortical midline structures (CMS).[32] The CMS are involved in self-referential thinking,[32–34] including SIT.[34,35] The CMS are involved in emotional processing.[36,37] Thus these regions may serve as the neurobiological link between self-referential thinking and emotional dysregulation in mood disorders, and may be particularly relevant to the effects of mindfulness. Numerous studies suggest that mindfulness alters CMS activation,[7] therefore modifying CMS function may be a key mechanism of mindfulness practices.

The anterior insula is important for explicit subjective awareness,[38–40] and thus has been thought to be important for mindful awareness. Mindfulness training decreases CMS activation and increases activation of the insula.[7] This finding suggests that shifting neural processing from the CMS to the insula is likely an important neurobiological mechanism associated with the change from narrative to experiential self-reference.

The lateral prefrontal cortex (PFC) plays a role in executive behavioral control[41] and emotional regulation[42,43] through modulation of the amygdala response.[44] There is evidence that meditation increases activation of the lateral PFC,[7] augmenting emotional control and thereby reducing symptoms of emotional overreactivity (see the article elsewhere in this issue for more discussion of emotion regulatory pathways).

RESEARCH REVIEW OF MINDFULNESS INTERVENTIONS

An extensive body of literature supporting the effectiveness of mindfulness interventions for the alleviation of psychiatric symptoms has been reviewed elsewhere,[7] and a brief synopsis is provided here. It has been pointed out[45–47] that many studies of mindfulness-based interventions have substantial methodological limitations. One of the most significant criticisms concerns the lack of high-quality, randomized controlled studies that use adequate comparators.[47] Other limitations include absence of follow-up measures, small sample size, reliance on self-report instruments, and a variety of differences across interventions.[45,47,48]

With these limitations in mind, studies suggest[7] that several psychological and physiologic benefits may be associated with mindfulness practices and meditation. Such benefits include better attention, enhanced self-compassion, decreased ruminative thinking, reduced cortisol levels, improved immune function, lower blood pressure, attenuated emotional reactivity, and enhanced cognition.

Studies indicate that MBSR is effective in relieving depressive and anxiety symptoms, including post-traumatic stress disorder. MBSR has been shown to decrease pain and increase pain coping, improve insomnia, enhance general mental health, and improve psychological functioning among individuals with a variety of medical disorders. However, a meta-analysis concluded that MBSR provides only relatively small effects on the reduction of depression, anxiety, and psychological distress in people with chronic medical illness.[49] Furthermore, 2 rigorous studies found benefit equivalent to, but not better than, an active control condition.[50,51]

With regard to MBCT, the strongest evidence is for relapse prevention in unipolar illness,[46,52–58] particularly among those with 3 or more prior episodes. Furthermore, MBCT offers protection against relapse equal to that of maintenance antidepressant pharmacotherapy.[7,57] In addition, evidence suggests efficacy for those experiencing a current episode and for those in remission.[59,60] Finally, at least 1 study indicates that MBCT is as effective as cognitive-behavioral therapy in the treatment of current depression.[55]

Other studies indicate that this intervention may also be beneficial for bipolar disorder, generalized anxiety disorder, panic disorder, hypochondriasis, and social phobia.[7]

POTENTIAL RISKS AND ADVERSE EFFECTS

Very little is currently known about the potential adverse effects of MBSR and MBCT. Although the risk of negative effects is likely low, further study is needed. One potential negative consequence is using a mindfulness intervention instead of a more effective treatment. Therefore clinicians should at present recommend MBSR and MBCT only as adjunctive interventions.

TREATMENT GUIDELINES FOR MBSR AND MBCT

Enough evidence exists to develop some general guidelines for the use of MBSR and MBCT in clinical practice as adjunctive interventions for mood and anxiety disorders. MBCT is strongly recommended as an adjunctive intervention for maintenance treatment/relapse prevention in unipolar illness. This intervention may also be considered as an adjunctive approach for acute and residual unipolar symptoms. Both MBSR and MBCT are recommended as adjunctive treatments for anxiety symptoms. Furthermore, MBSR is beneficial for pain management and general psychological health/stress management among those with medical or psychiatric illness as well as healthy individuals.

Only limited evidence is available to guide decisions about which patients are most likely to benefit from mindfulness-based interventions. Thus there is some risk of referring individuals for mindfulness who are not good candidates for this approach. A few studies provide some guidance.

Patient preference is important, and it is prudent to only refer patients who are relatively enthusiastic about trying mindfulness.[50,61] The level of commitment to an ongoing meditation practice is also relevant because evidence suggests that meditation-associated changes in brain function may require extensive practice.[62] Furthermore, considerable research indicates that greater meditation practice is associated with more improvement on some outcome measures.[56,63–65] Therefore, the most important considerations may be desire to try mindfulness and willingness to engage in a regular practice of meditation.

One approach is to have a relatively detailed discussion about mindfulness-based interventions with patients being considered for referral. This conversation could include an explanation of the concept of mindfulness and a brief mention of the evidence for effectiveness. **Box 1** provides some sample text to use when explaining mindfulness. Most importantly, such an exchange could provide the clinician with an idea of a patient's level of interest and motivation. **Box 2** provides some sample text to use when assessing patient interest and motivation.

Another important consideration for clinicians is finding mindfulness providers to refer to. One resource is the University of Massachusetts Center for Mindfulness Web site, which provides a list of MBSR providers by area (http://w3.umassmed.edu/MBSR/public/searchmember.aspx). For clinicians who may be interested in obtaining training to become providers of mindfulness interventions, information is available at the University of Massachusetts Center for Mindfulness Web site as well as the Center for Mindfulness at University of California San Diego Web site (http://health.ucsd.edu/specialties/mindfulness/Pages/default.aspx).

Box 1
Sample text for explaining mindfulness and meditation to patients

1. Mindfulness is nonjudgmental awareness of the sensations, thoughts, and emotions of the present moment.

2. In contrast to mindful awareness, the "autopilot" state of mind occurs when attention is focused on thoughts about the past or future and there is a sense of being carried away by one's cognitions and emotions. We spend most of our time with our minds on autopilot.

3. Autopilot can cause problems because not only are we caught up in our thoughts and emotions, but also our thinking can sometimes make us feel worse. For example, if we are feeling pain we experience the suffering from the pain, but if we start thinking about how bad it is and how long it may last, we increase the suffering.

4. When we are mindfully aware, we can have some distance from our thoughts and feelings. We can see them as transient phenomena that come and go like clouds in the sky. Having this space can decrease the effect our thoughts and feelings have, and give us the opportunity to see things more clearly.

5. Meditation involves focusing our attention on something, such as the physical sensations of breathing. During mindfulness meditation, moment-by-moment awareness is focused on sensations, thoughts, and emotions.

Box 2
Sample text to assess interest and motivation for mindfulness-based interventions

1. Does the concept of mindfulness make sense to you?

2. Are you interested in learning how to do mindfulness meditation?

3. Would you be willing to commit to attending an 8-week mindfulness class for approximately 2 hours per week?

4. Would you be willing to practice mindfulness meditation on your own 6 out of 7 days per week during the 8-week class?

WORKING WITH PATIENTS RECEIVING MINDFULNESS TRAINING

In addition to referring patients to mindfulness interventions, clinicians can support patients who are enrolled in a mindfulness class, such as MBSR or MBCT. To do so it is helpful to have a basic understanding of the intervention. The following is focused on MBCT, because it specifically targets psychiatric disorders. However, many aspects of MBSR are similar. MBCT is taught as a class rather than as a therapy group. It is highly experiential, and a large portion of class time is spent practicing mindfulness meditation in a group format. **Table 1** provides an overview of an 8-week MBCT course.[5] In addition to the topics listed in the table, all sessions include meditation practice as a group, and all except the first include homework review and discussion. **Table 2** describes the mindfulness meditation practices taught in MBCT.[5] For a complete description of an MBCT course, readers are referred to the book by Segal and colleagues,[5] the investigators who developed MBCT.

Table 1
Overview of an 8-week mindfulness-based cognitive therapy course

Session	Key Topics
Week 1	The mental states of "autopilot" and "mindfulness" First-hand experience of mindfulness: the raisin exercise Mindfulness practice: body scan
Week 2	Relationship between thoughts and emotions Awareness of pleasant events Mindfulness practice: sitting meditation
Week 3	Mindfulness practice: 3-minute breathing space Mindfulness practice: mindful stretching and walking Awareness of unpleasant events
Week 4	Automatic thoughts (autopilot) can lead to emotional distress Practice of meditation techniques learned previously
Week 5	Sitting meditation focusing on a difficult or stressful situation
Week 6	Thoughts are not facts Using the 3-minute breathing space in stressful situations
Week 7	Relationships between daily activities and depression Generate list of pleasure/mastery activities Identifying relapse triggers
Week 8	Course review Keeping a long-term meditation practice going

Data from Segal ZV, Williams JM, Teasdale JD. Mindfulness-based cognitive therapy for depression: a new approach to preventing relapse. New York: Guilford Press; 2002.

Table 2 Mindfulness practices of mindfulness-based cognitive therapy		
Practice	**Description**	**Purpose**
Raisin exercise	Participants eat a raisin slowly and focus awareness on sensations	First-hand experience of mindfulness
Body scan	Participants focus attention and awareness on a specific region of the body (eg, left foot) and then shift attention to another region	Learning a mindfulness practice to use on an ongoing basis
Sitting meditation	Attention is focused on the breath, body sensations, or thoughts and emotions	Learning to practice mindfulness and use as an ongoing practice
Walking and stretching meditation	Attention is focused on the physical sensations of movement and the breath	A practice to use on an ongoing basis
Three-minute breathing space	One first takes stock of his/her current situation. What's going on? What am I thinking and feeling? Attention is then focused on the breath for about a minute followed by a minute of focusing attention on bodily sensations	A short meditation to use on an ongoing basis, whenever one experiences unpleasant emotions or stress. The aim is to shift from the mental state of autopilot to mindfulness

Data from Segal ZV, Williams JM, Teasdale JD. Mindfulness-based cognitive therapy for depression: a new approach to preventing relapse. New York: Guilford Press; 2002.

One important way to support patients taking a mindfulness course is to encourage the development of a consistent daily practice of mindfulness meditation. There can be many barriers to daily practice, such as finding the time to practice and psychological resistance. With regard to making time for practice, most people do best if they have a specific time every day that is set aside for meditation. Often, first thing in the morning or last thing at night before bed works best. Encouraging patients to stick with their practice can be an important way for clinicians to support learning mindfulness skills.

SUMMARY

An expanding body of literature now exists that documents investigations of MBCT and MBSR, although some studies suffer from methodological limitations. However, these interventions show considerable promise and their clinical use is currently warranted. In particular, MBCT is recommended as an adjunctive treatment for unipolar depression. Both MBSR and MBCT have efficacy as adjunctive interventions for anxiety symptoms. MBSR is beneficial for general psychological health and pain management.

REFERENCES

1. Walsh R, Shapiro SL. The meeting of meditative disciplines and Western psychology: a mutually enriching dialogue. Am Psychol 2006;61(3):227–39.
2. Brown KW, Ryan RM. The benefits of being present: mindfulness and its role in psychological well-being. J Pers Soc Psychol 2003;84(4):822–48.

3. Kabat-Zinn J. Coming to our senses. New York: Hyperion; 2005.
4. Kabat-Zinn J. Full catastrophe living: using the wisdom of your body and mind to face stress, pain, and illness fifteenth anniversary edition. New York: Bantam Dell; 2005.
5. Segal ZV, Williams JM, Teasdale JD. Mindfulness-based cognitive therapy for depression: a new approach to preventing relapse. New York: Guilford Press; 2002.
6. Salmon P, Sephton S, Weissbecker I, et al. Mindfulness meditation in clinical practice. Cognit Behav Pract 2004;11(4):434–46.
7. Marchand WR. Mindfulness-based stress reduction, mindfulness-based cognitive therapy, and Zen meditation for depression, anxiety, pain, and psychological distress. J Psychiatr Pract 2012;18(4):233–52.
8. Mor N, Winquist J. Self-focused attention and negative affect: a meta-analysis. Psychol Bull 2002;128(4):638–62.
9. Ingram RE. Self-focused attention in clinical disorders: review and a conceptual model. Psychol Bull 1990;107(2):156–76.
10. Northoff G. Psychopathology and pathophysiology of the self in depression—neuropsychiatric hypothesis. J Affect Disord 2007;104(1–3):1–14.
11. Gallagher II. Philosophical conceptions of the self: implications for cognitive science. Trends Cogn Sci 2000;4(1):14–21.
12. Smallwood J, Schooler JW. The restless mind. Psychol Bull 2006;132(6):946–58.
13. McKiernan KA, D'Angelo BR, Kaufman JN, et al. Interrupting the "stream of consciousness": an fMRI investigation. Neuroimage 2006;29(4):1185–91.
14. Sakamoto S. A longitudinal study of the relationship of self-preoccupation with depression. J Clin Psychol 1999;55(1):109–16.
15. Burwell RA, Shirk SR. Subtypes of rumination in adolescence: associations between brooding, reflection, depressive symptoms, and coping. J Clin Child Adolesc Psychol 2007;36(1):56–65.
16. Spasojevic J, Alloy LB. Rumination as a common mechanism relating depressive risk factors to depression. Emotion 2001;1(1):25–37.
17. Michalak J, Holz A, Teismann T. Rumination as a predictor of relapse in mindfulness-based cognitive therapy for depression. Psychol Psychother 2011; 84(2):230–6.
18. Teasdale JD. Emotional processing, three modes of mind and the prevention of relapse in depression. Behav Res Ther 1999;37(Suppl 1):S53–77.
19. Watkins E, Teasdale JD. Adaptive and maladaptive self-focus in depression. J Affect Disord 2004;82(1):1–8.
20. Rimes KA, Watkins E. The effects of self-focused rumination on global negative self-judgements in depression. Behav Res Ther 2005;43(12):1673–81.
21. Williams AD, Moulds ML. The impact of ruminative processing on the experience of self-referent intrusive memories in dysphoria. Behav Ther 2010;41(1): 38–45.
22. Lo CS, Ho SM, Hollon SD. The effects of rumination and depressive symptoms on the prediction of negative attributional style among college students. Cognit Ther Res 2010;34(2):116–23.
23. Watkins E. Adaptive and maladaptive ruminative self-focus during emotional processing. Behav Res Ther 2004;42(9):1037–52.
24. Shapiro SL, Carlson LE, Astin JA, et al. Mechanisms of mindfulness. J Clin Psychol 2006;62(3):373–86.
25. Goldin PR, Gross JJ. Effects of mindfulness-based stress reduction (MBSR) on emotion regulation in social anxiety disorder. Emotion 2010;10(1):83–91.

26. Delgado LC, Guerra P, Perakakis P, et al. Treating chronic worry: psychological and physiological effects of a training programme based on mindfulness. Behav Res Ther 2010;48(9):873–82.
27. Brown KW, Goodman RJ, Inzlicht M. Dispositional mindfulness and the attenuation of neural responses to emotional stimuli. Soc Cogn Affect Neurosci 2013; 8(1):93–9.
28. Robins CJ, Keng SL, Ekblad AG, et al. Effects of mindfulness-based stress reduction on emotional experience and expression: a randomized controlled trial. J Clin Psychol 2012;68(1):117–31.
29. Taylor VA, Grant J, Daneault V, et al. Impact of mindfulness on the neural responses to emotional pictures in experienced and beginner meditators. Neuroimage 2011;57(4):1524–33.
30. Kemeny ME, Foltz C, Cavanagh JF, et al. Contemplative/emotion training reduces negative emotional behavior and promotes prosocial responses. Emotion 2012; 12(2):338–50.
31. Hill CL, Updegraff JA. Mindfulness and its relationship to emotional regulation. Emotion 2012;12(1):81–90.
32. Northoff G, Bermpohl F. Cortical midline structures and the self. Trends Cogn Sci 2004;8(3):102–7.
33. Northoff G, Heinzel A, de Greck M, et al. Self-referential processing in our brain—a meta-analysis of imaging studies on the self. Neuroimage 2006;31(1):440–57.
34. McGuire PK, Paulesu E, Frackowiak RS, et al. Brain activity during stimulus independent thought. Neuroreport 1996;7(13):2095–9.
35. Mason MF, Norton MI, Van Horn JD, et al. Wandering minds: the default network and stimulus-independent thought. Science 2007;315(5810):393–5.
36. Grimm S, Boesiger P, Beck J, et al. Altered negative BOLD responses in the default-mode network during emotion processing in depressed subjects. Neuropsychopharmacology 2009;34(4):932–43.
37. Heinzel A, Bermpohl F, Niese R, et al. How do we modulate our emotions? Parametric fMRI reveals cortical midline structures as regions specifically involved in the processing of emotional valences. Brain Res Cogn Brain Res 2005;25(1):348–58.
38. Craig AD. Human feelings: why are some more aware than others? Trends Cogn Sci 2004;8(6):239–41.
39. Critchley HD, Wiens S, Rothstein P, et al. Neural systems supporting interoceptive awareness. Nat Neurosci 2004;7(2):189–95.
40. Craig AD. Significance of the insula for the evolution of human awareness of feelings from the body. Ann N Y Acad Sci 2011;1225:72–82.
41. Tanji J, Hoshi E. Role of the lateral prefrontal cortex in executive behavioral control. Physiol Rev 2008;88(1):37–57.
42. Ochsner KN, Bunge SA, Gross JJ, et al. Rethinking feelings: an FMRI study of the cognitive regulation of emotion. J Cogn Neurosci 2002;14(8):1215–29.
43. Phan KL, Fitzgerald DA, Nathan PJ, et al. Neural substrates for voluntary suppression of negative affect: a functional magnetic resonance imaging study. Biol Psychiatry 2005;57(3):210–9.
44. Herwig U, Baumgartner T, Kaffenberger T, et al. Modulation of anticipatory emotion and perception processing by cognitive control. Neuroimage 2007; 37(2):652–62.
45. Chiesa A, Serretti A. A systematic review of neurobiological and clinical features of mindfulness meditations. Psychol Med 2010;40(8):1239–52.
46. Chiesa A, Serretti A. Mindfulness based cognitive therapy for psychiatric disorders: a systematic review and meta-analysis. Psychiatry Res 2011;187(3):441–53.

47. Chiesa A, Malinowski P. Mindfulness-based approaches: are they all the same? J Clin Psychol 2011;67(4):404–24.
48. Fjorback LO, Arendt M, Ombol E, et al. Mindfulness-based stress reduction and mindfulness-based cognitive therapy—a systematic review of randomized controlled trials. Acta Psychiatr Scand 2011;124(2):102–19.
49. Bohlmeijer E, Prenger R, Taal E, et al. The effects of mindfulness-based stress reduction therapy on mental health of adults with a chronic medical disease: a meta-analysis. J Psychosom Res 2010;68(6):539–44.
50. Schmidt S, Grossman P, Schwarzer B, et al. Treating fibromyalgia with mindfulness-based stress reduction: results from a 3-armed randomized controlled trial. Pain 2011;152(2):361–9.
51. MacCoon DG, Imel ZE, Rosenkranz MA, et al. The validation of an active control intervention for mindfulness based stress reduction (MBSR). Behav Res Ther 2012;50(1):3–12.
52. Bondolfi G, Jermann F, der Linden MV, et al. Depression relapse prophylaxis with mindfulness-based cognitive therapy: replication and extension in the Swiss health care system. J Affect Disord 2010;122(3):224–31.
53. Godfrin KA, van Heeringen C. The effects of mindfulness-based cognitive therapy on recurrence of depressive episodes, mental health and quality of life: a randomized controlled study. Behav Res Ther 2010;48(8):738–46.
54. Kuyken W, Byford S, Taylor RS, et al. Mindfulness-based cognitive therapy to prevent relapse in recurrent depression. J Consult Clin Psychol 2008;76(6): 966–78.
55. Manicavasgar V, Parker G, Perich T. Mindfulness-based cognitive therapy vs cognitive behaviour therapy as a treatment for non-melancholic depression. J Affect Disord 2011;130(1–2):138–44.
56. Mathew KL, Whitford HS, Kenny MA, et al. The long-term effects of mindfulness-based cognitive therapy as a relapse prevention treatment for major depressive disorder. Behav Cogn Psychother 2010;38(5):561–76.
57. Segal ZV, Bieling P, Young T, et al. Antidepressant monotherapy vs sequential pharmacotherapy and mindfulness-based cognitive therapy, or placebo, for relapse prophylaxis in recurrent depression. Arch Gen Psychiatry 2010;67(12): 1256–64.
58. Piet J, Hougaard E. The effect of mindfulness-based cognitive therapy for prevention of relapse in recurrent major depressive disorder: a systematic review and meta-analysis. Clin Psychol Rev 2011;31(6):1032–40.
59. van Aalderen JR, Donders AR, Giommi F, et al. The efficacy of mindfulness-based cognitive therapy in recurrent depressed patients with and without a current depressive episode: a randomized controlled trial. Psychol Med 2012;42(5): 989–1001.
60. Finucane A, Mercer SW. An exploratory mixed methods study of the acceptability and effectiveness of mindfulness-based cognitive therapy for patients with active depression and anxiety in primary care. BMC Psychiatry 2006;6:14.
61. Preference Collaborative Review Group. Patients' preferences within randomised trials: systematic review and patient level meta-analysis. BMJ 2008;337: a1864.
62. Slagter HA, Lutz A, Greischar LL, et al. Mental training affects distribution of limited brain resources. PLoS Biol 2007;5(6):e138.
63. Rosenzweig S, Greeson JM, Reibel DK, et al. Mindfulness-based stress reduction for chronic pain conditions: variation in treatment outcomes and role of home meditation practice. J Psychosom Res 2010;68(1):29–36.

64. Lengacher CA, Johnson-Mallard V, Post-White J, et al. Randomized controlled trial of mindfulness-based stress reduction (MBSR) for survivors of breast cancer. Psychooncology 2009;18(12):1261–72.

65. Carmody J, Baer RA. Relationships between mindfulness practice and levels of mindfulness, medical and psychological symptoms and well-being in a mindfulness-based stress reduction program. J Behav Med 2008;31(1):23–33.

Open Focus Attention Training

Lester G. Fehmi, PhD*, Susan B. Shor, LCSW

KEYWORDS

- Open focus attention • Attention to attention • Attention training • Dissolving pain
- Narrow focus • Neurofeedback • Alpha synchrony • Stress

KEY POINTS

- Open Focus is an attention training process which derives its efficacy from enhancing and alternately reducing brain wave activity and imagining the feeling of space.
- Neurofeedback training of brain synchrony and the deepening of the feeling of space create the benefits described in this article.
- Certain forms of attention can bring about the dissolution of sensory experience and pain.

INTRODUCTION AND BACKGROUND

The Open Focus attention training program described here emerged out of Les Fehmi's 1966 work as a postdoctoral student at The Brain Research Institute at UCLA. Fehmi observed that information processing in the visual systems of monkeys occurs as simultaneous, rather than sequential, events. This led to a search for other occasions in which synchrony or simultaneity occurred in the central nervous system. Alpha waves, high amplitude, midrange brain wave frequencies are associated with relaxed alertness and were known to be synchronous across brain locations. Synchronous waves peak and trough at the same time. Alpha synchrony is associated with autonomic nervous system balance, enabling the nervous system to operate more fluidly and effortlessly. Alpha synchrony supports stress reduction, increased intellectual and physical proficiency, and physical and emotional pain dissolution. Dr Joe Kamiya at the University of California showed that student subjects could recognize when they produced alpha wave activity and suggested that it might be possible to learn how to control such activity.

Fehmi discovered how to produce increased amplitudes and durations of synchronous alpha. Practice over time was associated with positive changes: decreased anxiety, increased emotional intimacy, greater sense of ease, freedom, and fluidity.

Research on the ability of student subjects to increase alpha synchrony, later called brain wave biofeedback or neurofeedback, led to the discovery that controlling production of brain wave activity could alter physical, emotional, and intellectual functioning.

Princeton Biofeedback Centre, 317 Mount Lucas Road, Princeton, NJ 08540, USA
* Corresponding author.
E-mail address: lesfehmi@openfocus.com

Psychiatr Clin N Am 36 (2013) 153–162
http://dx.doi.org/10.1016/j.psc.2013.01.003
0193-953X/13/$ – see front matter © 2013 Elsevier Inc. All rights reserved.

Relaxation Doesn't Help Much

Relaxation is a by-product, not a cause, of alpha synchrony. Electroencephalogram (EEG) studies demonstrated that the then-known methods of relaxation training (eg, beautiful music, pleasant smells, guided relaxation imagery, hypnotic inductions, autogenic training, progressive muscle relaxation training) had no significant impact on production of synchronous alpha activity. However, when a 20-item visual relaxation inventory was used, 2 of the questions yielded a reliable impact on the alpha synchronous activity. Those 2 questions were the following:

1. "Can you imagine the space between your eyes?"
2. "Can you imagine the space between your ears?"

The word that appears in both is "space." The relevant variable is that they require attention to space. Attending to space, particularly to the feeling of space, increased production of synchronous alpha activity.

ATTENTION STYLE

With training, we can learn to move from attention styles that are narrow and objective, to ones that are more diffuse and immersed. Space is objectless and ubiquitous, and attending to it naturally opens our attention and encourages immersion. This concept led to an interest in attention to attention.

Attention is a fundamental behavior that reflects in brain wave activity, physiologic arousal, and emotional responses. **Fig. 1** shows 4 continua of attention:

1. The first moves left from center toward increasing diffuse attention
2. The second moves right from the center toward increasing narrow attention

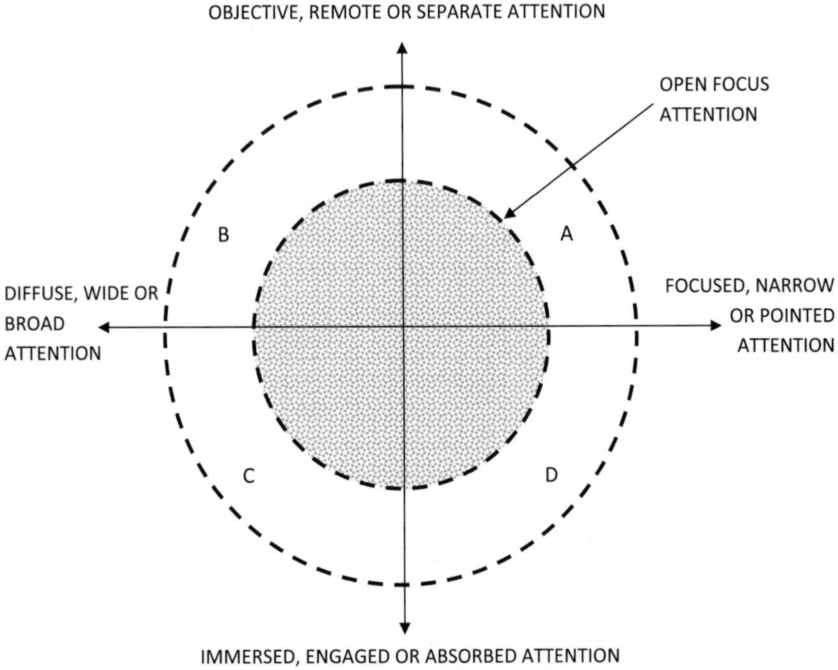

Fig. 1. Individual attention types. A, B, C, D: Sectors represent attention style combinations. Central area represents open focus attention.

3. The third moves up from the center toward increasing objective attention
4. The fourth moves down from the center toward increasing immersed attention

These continua are at right angles, indicating independence from one another, which allows for combinations of attention. The dotted circles indicate that it is possible to engender all of these attentional styles equally and simultaneously, creating a comprehensive style of attention called Open Focus.

Understanding and practicing the various attention styles has clinical implications. **Table 1** shows that each attention combination is reflected in different behaviors, EEG patterns, and physiologic arousal levels.

Table 1
Styles of attention. Each attentional style, illustrated with examples, has particular effects on the nervous system with associated EEG patterns

	Diffuse-Immersed	Diffuse-Objective	Narrow-Immersed	Narrow-Objective
Examples	Meditation. With mind unselfconscious and body at rest. Most rapid normalization. Sleep.	Panoramic view in a "symphony of sensory experience." Objective sensations hang suspended in the midst of a diffuse awareness of space. Playing in a band.	Immersed in enjoyment, amplified by a narrow focus to intensify and savor experience. Enraptured thinker. Deep massage recipient.	Lion stalking its prey. Emergency. College examination. Obsessing on work to narrow focus away from (deny) an emotional problem. Self-conscious mind and body. Highly toned.
Effects	Parasympathetic nervous system dominance. Low arousal. Mostly right brain dominant. Drifting into sleep.	Relative sympathetic and parasympathetic balance. Moderate arousal. Relative left-right hemisphere balance. Relaxed alert.	Relative sympathetic and parasympathetic balance. Moderate arousal. Left-right hemisphere balance. Relaxed alert.	Sympathetic nervous system dominance. High arousal-adrenaline. Mostly left brain dominance. Extreme fight or flight.
EEG	Low frequencies dominant. Increased amplitude. Increased whole brain activity.	Middle frequencies dominant in alpha. Moderate whole brain synchrony.	Middle frequencies dominant in alpha. Moderate whole brain synchrony.	High frequencies increase: high beta and gamma. Reduced amplitude overall. Reduce whole brain activity synchrony.

Low frequencies, below 8 Hz, delta and theta; Middle frequencies, 8–15 Hz, alpha; High frequencies, 15–60 Hz, high beta and gamma.
Abbreviation: EEG, electroencephalogram.

The Significance of Attention Styles

Space is objectless and ubiquitous, and attending to it in a certain way opens our attention and encourages immersion. We have the ability to consciously change how we pay attention to space:

- We can broaden our attention to space, thereby increasing the diffusion of attention to include space and all the objects in it, in every sensory modality.
- We can exclude space, thereby narrowing and objectifying our attention to one or more objects.
- We can immerse our attention into space and objects.
- We can distance ourselves from space and objects, becoming more separate.
- Or we can do all of these things at once in Open Focus attention.

Each of these choices in how we attend is reflected in brain wave activity. Synchronous alpha is produced in greater abundance when we pay attention to space in all the different styles at once, so that we are immersed and objective, and narrow and diffuse at the same time. **Fig. 1** is a diagram of attentional styles.

Understanding and practicing the various attention styles depicted in **Fig. 1** has clinical implications. **Table 1** shows that each attention combination is associated with different behaviors, EEG patterns, and physiologic arousal levels. With practice, one can learn to access all of the attention styles depicted in **Fig. 1** and **Table 1**.

The value of practicing attention training lies in the fact that it is possible to control arousal levels through the manipulation of attention styles. It is physiologically and psychologically important to maintain relatively stable levels of arousal. If our arousal levels are chronically low, we feel sleepy, lethargic, depressed, and do not function optimally. If arousal levels are chronically high, we are hypervigilant, stressed, anxious, and behavior is not optimal. In the mid range of arousal, for most tasks, we are performing evenly at peak levels. In **Fig. 2** the simultaneous combination of all attention styles (Open Focus) is illustrated by the intersecting dotted and dashed curves, which produce ideal arousal levels.

DISSOLVING PAIN

The reduction of stress and resultant optimum functioning are important benefits of attention training. Using attention styles that lead the user to immerse himself or herself into the feeling of pain, while at the same time remaining in a diffuse attention mode, both of which are permeated by space, results in dissolution of pain. Immersion into and diffusion of pain and space encourages the production of synchronous alpha activity, which reduces stress and dissolves pain.

Destroying the Subject-object World

It is through the production of synchronous brain wave activity, coexisting with asynchronous activity, that the world of objects is created and destroyed. The sine waves in **Fig. 3** show that the top 2 waves are asynchronous with one other, whereas the second and third sine waves are perfectly synchronous. The third and fourth waves are half in and half out of phase.

When one part of the brain is out of phase with another, then something is perceived as an object. When all parts are in phase, one is immersed, at one with the experience. There is no differentiation between subject and object. To objectify something, the phase relationship changes such that the object is in one phase while the awareness is out of phase. In this regard, the visual system has been studied the most. For example, the occipital cortex is usually out of phase with the frontal cortex (including

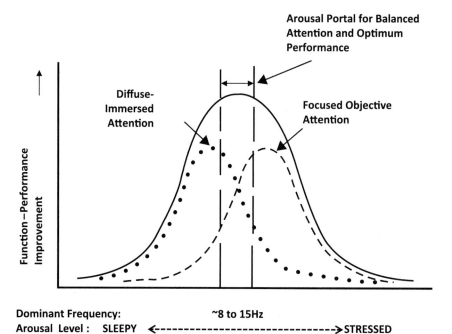

Fig. 2. Proposed relationship between arousal Performance, and EEG dominant frequencies and attention style as they impact function - Performance.

the prefrontal cortex). Being out of phase enables images (the object image) formed in the occipital cortex to be witnessed (perceived) in the frontal cortex.

The Role of Phase in Dissolving Pain

Asynchronous brain activity gives rise to objective experience. Objective experience is represented by islands of asynchronous activity (relative to the activity of the subject). These islands of objectivity, of asynchrony, dissolve when the process of objectification ceases and synchrony is resumed. The process of objectification gives way to the experience of union and to "no-time," and unselfconsciousness.

Asynchronous brain wave activity can be converted into synchronous activity by adopting an attention to space that is immersed and diffused; by attending to the space in and around and through the "object," we can convert the asynchronous activity of the "object" into synchronous activity of the "subject." This causes the islands of asynchronous activity to dissolve. Thus, the "pain" dissolves. Using the guiding exercises presented later in this article, any experience can be dissolved. See the **Dissolving Pain exercise**.

The subject and the object exist in 2 dominant wave frequencies that are close, but not quite equal to one another. When they meet, a new phase relationship is created with the self. Simple awareness occurs when we are not aware of our awareness. Simple awareness allows unconscious behaviors, such as riding a bicycle. It is possible to engage in an activity, such as driving a car, and to realize after some time that one was driving without self-awareness. Simple awareness allows us to function.

When the self approaches and immerses in the object, all 3 (subject, object, and self) become one, such that there is no simple awareness and no awareness of

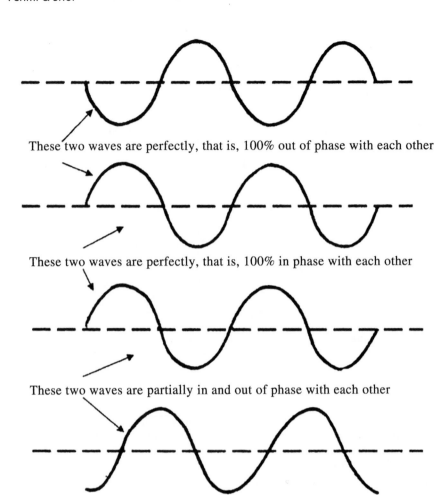

These two waves are perfectly, that is, 100% out of phase with each other

These two waves are perfectly, that is, 100% in phase with each other

These two waves are partially in and out of phase with each other

Fig. 3. Examples of sine wave phase relations.

awareness. The use of immersion in space during open focus meditation enables this state of nonawareness to emerge. When, for example, a particular pain is chosen as the object, the degree to which the immersion in space is successful becomes evident in the degree to which the experience of the pain is diluted, becomes "thinner" and more diffuse, and spreads into the other parts of the brain until it is no longer distinguishable as a separate experience. Thus, as the brain wave activity becomes more in-phase, at one phase, there is no experience of pain.

Dissolving Pain in the Clinic

Learning how to dissolve pain is therapeutic. Furthermore, it enables clients to address and engage with their pain, knowing that they can dissolve the pain as they go along. Open Focus considers anxiety, depression, and many other symptoms to be forms of pain, requiring only that individuals be able to locate their emotions as physical sensations and then move toward and immerse their attention into those sensations. Relief comes as they learn to diffuse their attention into the space the pain occupies and the space around the pain.

A series of recorded Open Focus Training exercises can be practiced to improve attentional flexibility. These are effective, in inducing alpha synchrony across the brain. Through the training of attentional flexibility, the user can reduce stress levels, produce optimum arousal levels, and effectively dissolve unwanted sensations, such as pain. All this is done by attending to how we attend, by recognizing that we can make attentional choices, and can flexibly manipulate these choices, selecting the appropriate attention styles for the situation at hand. The following case illustrates the principles of Open Focus treatment for emotional pain.

OPEN FOCUS TRAINING EXERCISES

The following scripts of 2 Open Focus training exercises can be practiced in sequence or separately:

Before we start, please sit up in your chair with your hands resting in your lap and, if you feel comfortable, close your eyes. You will be asked to imagine feeling sensations and their absence. Imagining is like pretending. Don't try hard. Just let your imagination do all the work.

Space is like the air in the room. There is space all around you, in front of you, behind you, to the left of you, to the right of you, and above and below you. Space is also inside you, even though it doesn't seem that way. So when I ask you to let yourself feel space inside and outside your body, just do the best you can. It is like imagining you are a balloon and you can feel the space inside and outside at the same time.

It is easier to feel space when your eyes are closed. Let yourself feel the space in that part of your body mentioned in the exercise as best you can without trying. I will let 10 seconds go by before asking you what it would feel like to feel another space in your body.

You might be interested to know that the more we feel space, the more our body and brain relaxes its grip on itself. The more relaxed we are the better we feel, the happier we are, and the more we can pay attention effortlessly. So that's why the exercise asks you to feel lots of space, space inside your body and outside your body.

Now, please move on to the first exercise called General Space Exercise.

General space exercise

Can you imagine feeling comfortable in a chair?

Can you imagine feeling the space in the whole room you are in?

Can you imagine feeling the presence of your thumbs?

Can you imagine feeling your thumbs more clearly if you move them slowly?

Can you imagine feeling the presence of your index fingers?

Can you imagine feeling the presence of your thumbs and index fingers simultaneously?

Can you imagine feeling and now also the space around?

Can you imagine feeling and also the space they occupy?

Can you imagine feeling the continuity of space through your fingers?

Can you imagine feeling the space between the thumb and index finger of each hand?

Can you imagine feeling the space these fingers are moving though very slowly?

Can you imagine feeling the space between these fingers as they widen and narrow?

Can you imagine feeling the sense of presence of your remaining fingers?

Can you imagine feeling the space around and between them?

Can you imagine feeling the space they occupy?

Can you imagine feeling the continuity of space through all your fingers?

Can you imagine feeling the continuity of space through your hands and fingers?

Can you imagine feeling a detailed experience of space surrounding and permeating other body parts until all are simultaneously included?

Can you imagine feeling that you are bathing in space?

Can you imagine feeling that you are resting in space?

Can you imagine feeling that you practice this exercise at least twice daily?

Dissolving pain exercise

- Can you imagine sitting comfortably in your chair?
- Can you imagine feeling the space above and below your body?
- Can you imagine feeling the space to the left and to the right of your body?
- Can you imagine feeling the space in front of your body and behind your body?
- Can you imagine feeling the space in the whole room?
- Can you imagine feeling the space beyond the room extending in every direction?
- Can you remember what it is like to feel the space inside your body and the space outside your body at the same time?
- Can you imagine feeling space so intimately that it feels like you are space?
- Can you imagine feeling your hands and arms filled with and surrounded by space?
- Can you imagine feeling your feet and legs filled with and surrounded by space?
- Can you imagine feeling your lower body from the waist down filled with space and surrounded by space?
- Can you imagine feeling your upper body, up to your neck, filled and surrounded by space?
- Can you imagine feeling your head and neck filled with space and surrounded by space?
- Can you imagine feeling your whole body filled with space? Can you imagine feeling the space around your body: in front of your body, behind your body, to the left of your body, to the right of your body, below your body, and above your body?
- Can you imagine as you feel your whole body filled with space and surrounded by space, you can also imagine that you are feeling space everywhere, inside and outside your body at the same time?
- Can you imagine bathing in a vast space?
- Now that you are feeling all that space, can you notice if you are feeling any pain, like a stomach ache or a headache, or tension or if you are feeling any unpleasant emotion, such as worry, anger, insecurity, boredom, fear, nervousness, disappointment, sleepiness. If you are feeling a chronic emotion that you don't want, notice where you feel it in your body. You may never have thought that an emotion could be felt in the body. You might think that feelings are only in your mind, but if you feel into your body, you can also find that some emotions that last for a while and that you don't like, such as worry, for example, are really felt in your body.
- When I feel anxiety, which I feel as worry or a nervous feeling, I feel it sometimes in my chest and sometimes in my throat. When you can find an emotion like that somewhere in your body, you can learn to dissolve it. So let's use either an emotion or vague feeling that you don't like, which you have found in your body, or a physical pain, like a headache or stomach

ache. Use whichever is stronger and let's dissolve it. The feeling we are going to dissolve, whatever its nature, will be called your "pain."

- Can you imagine feeling your pain and giving it a number on a 10 scale? If it is very strong and you feel you can't stand it anymore, give it a 10. If there is no pain give it a zero. Assign numbers in between for intensities of an intermediate level.
- Can you imagine feeling the space inside your body and around your body and in the room and beyond? Can you imagine bathing in that space? As you continue to do that can you also imagine feeling the pain in the center of your attention?
- Can you imagine feeling that your pain has a shape and a size, like a ball or a pea?
- Can you imagine feeling the pain more?
- Can you imagine feeling the height and width and depth of your pain?
- Can you imagine feeling the space that your pain occupies?
- Can you imagine that you can feel your pain is a cloud of particles, floating in space, permeated by space?
- Can you imagine that you can feel your pain filled with space and surrounded by space?
- While you are feeling the space in the whole room and the space inside your body, can you imagine feeling the space around your pain and the space that your pain occupies? As you are immersing yourself in the pain, can you imagine your pain spreading in every direction?
- Can you imagine feeling what's left of the pain even more softly and intimately and continue to let is spread?
- Can you imagine as you feel the pain even more, you can imagine also bathing in it as you would in a warm bath?
- Can you imagine basking in the pain as you would if you were taking a sun bath?
- Can you imagine melting into the pain?
- Can you imagine dissolving into the pain?
- If the pain has disappeared, then can you imagine feeling into where your pain was and then feel for any remaining pain that is still there, like tension or numbness or emptiness or other feeling. Can you imagine feeling into that new or remaining pain until it dissipates also?
- Can you notice what number your pain is? If it is a zero, you can stop the exercise. If some of the original pain is still there, see if you can merge into it until it dissolves completely.

CLINICAL GUIDELINES

In deciding which clients are likely to benefit from Open Focus, the following factors can be useful. First, is the client interested and motivated enough. Those with intractable chronic pain that has not responded to standard treatments tend to be the most highly motivated. Also, many people simply do not want to take prescription analgesics or opiates because they are concerned about adverse affects, habituation, or addiction. Open Focus has been particularly beneficial for certain populations, for example, military veterans and patients with cancer.

Adverse Reactions and Contraindications

One concern of a few individuals is that the attention of space in Open Focus Training could cause patients with schizophrenia to dissociate. In the authors' experience (L.G.F. and S.B.S.), Open Focus training reduces identity breaks. This is especially so when they learn to merge and separate alternately. The authors have treated a handful of patients with schizophrenia who all improved. The authors consider dissociation and related disorders, such as posttraumatic stress disorder, to be disorders of attention.

SUMMARY

Clinicians who learn Open Focus meditation acquire a valuable skill that can be used for their own self-healing as well as in teaching clients how to dissolve pain as they work through their physical and emotional issues. Alternatively, clients can use recorded CD training or online webinars to teach themselves. This is more likely to be successful when the clinician explains the process, monitors patient compliance, and motivates the patient to practice enough to become proficient in attention training and to obtain the fullest benefits.

FURTHER READINGS

Fehmi LG. Multichannel EEG phase synchrony training and verbally guided attention training for disorders of attention. In: Evans JR, editor. Handbook of neurofeedback. Binghampton: Haworth Press, Inc; 2007. p. 301–20.

Fehmi LG, Atkins J, Lindsey DB. The electrophysiological correlates of perceptual masking in monkeys. Exp Brain Res 1969;7:299–316.

Fehmi LG, Fritz G. Open focus: the attentional foundation of health and well-being. Somatics 1980;24–30.

Fehmi LG, Robbins J. Dissolving pain: simple brain-training exercises for overcoming chronic pain. Boston: Trumpeter Books; 2010.

Fehmi LG, Robbins J. Mastering our brain's electrical rhythm. Cerebrum 2001;3(3): 55–67.

Fehmi LG, Robbins J. Sweet Surrender. In: Goleman D, editor. Measuring the Immeasurable: The Scientific Case for Spirituality. Boulder: Sounds True, Inc; 2008. p. 231–42.

Fehmi LG, Robbins J. The open focus brain: harnessing the power of attention to heal mind and body. Boston: Trumpeter Books, An imprint of Shambhala Publications, Inc; 2007 (Forthcoming in translation: German, Chinese, French, Korean, Dutch, Mainland China).

Fehmi LG, Sundor A. The effects of electrode placement upon EEG biofeedback training: the monopolar-bipolar controversy. Int J Psychosom 1989;36:23–33.

Larsen S. The neurofeedback solution: how to treat autism, ADHD, anxiety, brain injury, stroke, PTSD, and more. Rochester: Healing Arts Press; 2012.

McKnight JT, Fehmi LG. Attention and neurofeedback synchrony training: clinical results and their significance. J Neurother 2001;5(1):45–61.

Robbins J. A symphony in the brain: the evolution of the new brain wave biofeedback. New York: Atlantic Monthly Press; 2000.

Sichel A, Fehmi LG, Goldstein D. Positive outcome with neurofeedback treatment in a case of mind autism. J Neurother 1995;1(1):60–4.

Sugerman AA, Tarter RE, Fehmi LG. EEG biofeedback, multichannel synchrony training, and attention. In: Sugarman AA, Tarter RE, editors. Expanding Dimensions of Consciousness. New York: Springer Publishing Company, Inc; 1978. p. 155–82.

Valdez MR. A program of stress management in a college setting. Psychother Priv Pract 1988;6(2):43–54.

Neurofeedback

An Emerging Technology for Treating Central Nervous System Dysregulation

Stephen Larsen, PhD[a,b], Leslie Sherlin, PhD[c,d,e,f,g],*

KEYWORDS

- Neurofeedback • QEEG • PTSD • ADHD • Seizure • Treatment

KEY POINTS

- Neurofeedback, a subspecialization of biofeedback, is based on learning theory (eg, classical and operant conditioning).
- Neurofeedback is best administered by a qualified or licensed professional who has received training in one or more subspecializations.
- Neurofeedback is often used in combination with other treatments such as medication or psychotherapy.
- Neurofeedback is efficacious for epilepsy, Attention Deficit Hyperactivity Disorder (ADHD), and anxiety disorders.
- Neurofeedback is probably efficacious for traumatic brain injury, alcoholism and other substance abuse, insomnia, and optimal/peak performance.
- Evidence of efficacy for neurofeedback monotherapy is insufficient for depression, autism, Post Traumatic Stress Disorder (PTSD), and tinnitus, although outcomes are positive in the limited available studies.

BACKGROUND AND CLINICAL APPLICATIONS

Biofeedback is a method of treatment in which patients are trained to become aware of and learn to control their own physiology to improve physical and psychological health. Neurofeedback, a subspecialization of biofeedback, also called electroencephalogram (EEG) biofeedback, uses the patient's EEG as feedback to modify the brain's electrical activity patterns.[1] In contrast, other biofeedback modalities use physiologic measures, such as pulse, skin temperature, or heart rate variability as

a Stone Mountain Center, 310 River Road Exd, New Paltz, NY 12561, USA; b SUNY, Ulster, Stone Ridge, NY, USA; c Neurotopia, Inc, Marina Del Rey, CA, USA; d Nova Tech EEG, Inc, 8503 East Keats Avenue, Mesa, AZ 85209, USA; e Arizona Brain Performance Center, Mesa, AZ, USA; f Southwest College of Naturopathic Medicine, Tempe, AZ, USA; g University of Phoenix, Phoenix, AZ, USA
* Corresponding author. 8503 East Keats Avenue, Mesa, AZ 85209.
E-mail address: lesliesherlin@mac.com

Psychiatr Clin N Am 36 (2013) 163–168
http://dx.doi.org/10.1016/j.psc.2013.01.005
0193-953X/13/$ – see front matter © 2013 Elsevier Inc. All rights reserved.

feedback to alter brain activity and physiologic functions. The history, research, and clinical effects of neurofeedback have been reviewed in-depth elsewhere.[2–4]

Classic conditioning of the human EEG, specifically the "alpha blocking response," was accomplished in France[5] and in the United States.[6] During the 1940s, Gibbs and Knott[7] noticed that the frequencies of brainwaves measured in Hertz (Hz), cycles per second, gradually increase through the life-cycle: slower brain waves, delta (0.5–3.5 Hz) and theta (4–7.5 Hz), predominate in infants and young children. These slower frequencies are associated with injury or functional immaturity in awake adults. Excessive slow wave activity was found to be associated with symptoms consistent with what is known today as ADHD.[8] By 1962, it was demonstrated that individuals could learn to modulate their own EEG through operant conditioning.[9] For a comprehensive review of the history connecting classic/operant conditioning to neurofeedback see Sherlin and colleagues.[3] The idea of volitional control over one's brain activity led to the theory that changing the EEG could lead to clinical improvements among patients with mental health diagnoses.

High-quality randomized controlled trials (RCTs) have shown significant benefits from neurotherapy, primarily in treatment of ADHD. Strehl and colleagues[10,11] conducted an RCT in which subjects received training in theta/beta neurofeedback or slow cortical potential neurofeedback. Both interventions showed positive and similar improvements in ADHD symptoms, which were sustained at 6-month follow-up[12]; Holtmann and colleagues completed an RCT of theta/beta neurofeedback versus a control group using Captain's Log training.[13] Both groups participated in attention training programs for the same amount of time. This study found a specific and clinically relevant improvement in impulsivity on a go-no go task only in the neurofeedback group. Parent rating scales indicated significant improvements in inattention, hyperactivity, and impulsivity. A multicenter double-blind RCT of 94 patients with ADHD found that treatment with neurofeedback resulted in significant improvements in subscales of attention and hyperactivity/impulsivity symptoms measured by an ADHD rating scale[14] and in reduction of the theta band EEG compared with no change in the control group given a credible sham attention training.[15] Postevaluation analysis of data from this sample demonstrated specificity of neurofeedback and reduced EEG theta power in the neurofeedback group but not in the control group.[16]

Seizure Disorders

M. Barry Sterman discovered that cats were able to become seizure resistant by learning to produce a particular morphological wave form in the low beta frequency range (12–15 Hz), called sensory motor rhythm, over the sensory motor cortex. The National Aeronautics and Space Administration contacted Sterman to investigate seizure activity in astronauts and service personnel exposed to monomethyl hydrazine, a highly volatile rocket-fuel additive. This investigation led to the development of neurofeedback protocols to control epilepsy.[17]

Attention-Deficit/Hyperactivity Disorder

Joel F. Lubar detected outcomes of increased calmness in those trained with neurofeedback for seizure disorders and postulated efficacy for the hyperkinesis and disorganization of ADHD, predominantly hyperactive-impulsive type.[18] Lubar found the EEG ratio of theta to beta waves at the vertex (CZ in the International 10-20 system) to be the most reliable indicator of attention problems and pioneered neurofeedback protocols for treating ADHD.[19] The characteristic pattern in ADHD, excess theta and insufficient beta (13–21 Hz), is associated with deficits in activation and occurs primarily in the frontal lobe. Neurofeedback training protocols that reduce theta and increase beta (eg, theta/beta ratio training) therefore positively affect ADHD symptoms. Subsequent research confirmed and extended his findings such that ADHD, both predominantly inattentive and combined types, became the best-documented disorder illustrating neurofeedback efficacy.[2,20,21]

Posttraumatic Stress Disorder

Earlier research in neurofeedback pertained to the development of treatment of PTSD in returning war veterans. Although the first protocols showed efficacy in trauma recovery by augmenting the 7-Hz range (theta), often the treatment experience vividly evoked the original trauma or retraumatized the patient. Peniston and Kulkosky[22] found that the addition of alpha (8–12 Hz) to the theta treatment produced a soothing, mitigating affect on the treatment experience, rendering it more tolerable. Although substantial recoveries were reported in Vietnam veterans with drug and alcohol addiction as well as PTSD, they were met with skepticism. The lack of double-blind RCTs left the treatment open to question and controversy.

NEUROFEEDBACK: METHODS AND MODALITIES

Neurofeedback training should begin with a clinical intake and baseline evaluation, which often includes a neuropsychological battery or at a minimum a computerized continuous performance test such as the test of variables of attention, integrated visual and auditory, and/or a Quantitative Electroencephalography (qEEG).

Quantitative Electroencephalograph

The qEEG is a screening instrument in which 19 to 21 sites on the International 10-20 system are measured by an EEG amplifier. The results are processed on a computer, which can display the raw EEG and use the fast Fourier transform to calculate the components of the complex waveform into discrete frequency ranges. This result shows the proportion of the various waveform frequencies such as delta, theta, alpha, beta, and gamma. The analysis provides the magnitude in microvolts and the power (microvolts squared) across frequencies (in hertz), as well as other spectral metrics. In contrast to routine EEG, qEEG entails additional computer processing, and the results are compared with a reference population of healthy individuals (presumed normative). This database comparison analysis is designed to reflect normalcy or abnormality of brain activity by calculating standard deviations from the normative sample. Connectivity measures, such as coherence, asymmetry, and phase, across the sites and across the hemispheres, provide additional information about brain processing.[4]

Normative population data are compiled into databases in a variety of software platforms for processing qEEG data. Some analysis software contains subscales or discriminant metrics that measure the likelihood of the client to be statistically similar to a population of individuals with a known diagnosis, such as traumatic brain injury (TBI), learning disabilities, depression, dementia, obsessive-compulsive disorder, ADHD, or schizophrenia.[23] qEEG-guided neurofeedback treatment is deemed to be a superior method for guiding protocols by most practitioners.[4] Some report that using qEEG analysis to choose treatment protocols may improve efficacy by 50%.[24] In addition, a 3-dimensional imaging technique called low-resolution electromagnetic brain tomography (LORETA) calculates the "inverse solution" and is used to localize the cortical origin of electrical activity in deeper brain structures based on surface electrodes. A higher-resolution version (in voxels) with a demonstrated zero localization error is called exact or eLORETA.[25]

qEEG Clinical Administration

Neurofeedback is usually administered in the clinician's office using at least 3 electrodes at active sites for training, reference, and ground. There may be more active electrodes (as many as 19) used for training, depending on the complexity of the protocol. The client is asked to produce a brain electrical event for which certain feedback effects occur, for example, turn a sound on or off, move the level of an on-screen thermometer or bar graph, or watch a movie that dims or turns off when the client is not performing the task but turns on bright and clear if the client is "on target" (**Box 1**).

Typically, appointments last between a half-hour and an hour, and it is generally agreed that the sessions are of higher quality if the clinician stays in the room to monitor activities and make adjustments as necessary.[4] The number of sessions required to produce long-lasting results varies. Some report that 30 to 40 sessions are needed,[26] whereas others observe that it depends on the type and severity of the disorder. For example, autism spectrum disorders or Asperger syndrome may require 40 to 60 sessions.[27] Some have reported that in some sudden onset or acute problems where the premorbid condition was good, 5 to 10 sessions may produce remission.[28]

MECHANISMS OF ACTION

The primary purpose of neurofeedback is to create learned changes in electrical activity of the brain that are linked to clinical symptoms or are associated with positive states (eg, optimal performance). Neurofeedback contributes to neural plasticity by addressing excesses and deficits in particular frequency bands that are corrected using inhibition or augmentation training, respectively.[29] Gunkelman and Johnstone[26] refer to the concept of "growth through utilization" as being analogous to building muscle mass by repeated exercises and suggest that the training process itself may contribute to the

---

Box 1
Neurofeedback methods

- *Operant conditioning or contingency-based neurofeedback:* the subject is asked to augment one frequency range and inhibit another.[4]

- *qEEG-guided training:* the frequencies selected for operant conditioning training are based on analysis of the multisite EEG assessment and quantified metrics.

- *Z-score training:* the training feedback is based on moving predetermined variables closer to zero standard deviations or "within normal limits" based on a reference population of qEEGs.[2]

- *Low-energy neurofeedback system (LENS):* this procedure is passive, in which the subject sits with eyes closed during radiofrequency electromagnetic stimulation, said to be little or no more intense than the signals emitted by most EEG amplifiers but using special protocols developed by OchsLabs. This very low intensity treatment (10–18 or 10–21 W/cm^2) is said to be effective with brief applications and shorter treatment times than conventional neurofeedback protocols.[2,28]

- *Slow cortical potentials (SCP) training:* operant conditioning volitional control of the SCP has shown efficacy in attention, migraine, and seizure disorders.[34–36]

- *Neurofield:* this procedure is both passive and active (has a feedback loop for operant conditioning). It uses electromagnetic frequencies (as does the LENS) but may also have feedback components, such as heart rate variability or Z-score neurofeedback responses to guide treatment.[2,26]

strengthening of synapses. A greater proportion of theta and alpha frequency bands localized frontally correspond to decreased perfusion (blood flow) as seen on positron emission tomography.[30] Correlations between blood flow and EEG findings help explain one way in which neurofeedback might influence the brain. For example, theta activity is associated with decreased blood perfusion and beta with increased blood perfusion. This result implies that correcting the excessive theta activity and deficits of beta seen in the central and frontal areas of the brain in ADHD contributes to improvement in perfusion in areas of impaired or sluggish brain function.[31]

CLINICAL CONSIDERATIONS IN NEUROFEEDBACK
Efficacy Ratings

Neurofeedback efficacy is graded on a 1 to 5 scale, where a rating of 1 or not empirically supported consists primarily of case studies or anecdotal reports. A rating of 5 indicates that the therapy has been found to be superior to a placebo in RCTs conducted at a minimum of 2 independent sites.

1. Areas where neurofeedback has been deemed efficacious (level 4) or efficacious and specific (level 5) are epilepsy, ADHD, and anxiety spectrum disorders.
2. Areas where neurofeedback has been deemed probably efficacious (level 3) include TBI, alcoholism/substance abuse, insomnia and optimal/peak performance.
3. Areas where evidence of efficacy is insufficient (level 2) include depressive disorders, autism, PTSD, and tinnitus. This lower rating of efficacy is due to the insufficient number of studies or the minimal sample sizes used in reported studies despite findings of positive outcomes.

Side Effects and Adverse Reactions

Any treatment method can cause harm, particularly when used injudiciously. Neurofeedback practitioners, in promoting their method as "holistic" and "noninvasive," may misrepresent its potential to cure serious illnesses or to destabilize patients who are precariously adapted. Practitioners can be naive or irresponsible in applying treatments that may be too intense, too long, or unlikely to succeed in particular conditions.[32] Sensitivity, overreactivity, or a precarious adaptation can predispose a patient to adverse reactions to neurofeedback sessions. Potential side effects include headache, nausea, dizziness, fatigue, agitation, cognitive interference, or destabilization.[33] These side effects are infrequent and usually resolve within a few hours.

Professional Regulation and Credentialing

No government body specifically regulates the licensure of neurofeedback practitioners. Professional credentials and/or licensure in a health profession is required for those who treat disorders described in the Diagnostic and Statistical Manual of Mental Disorders and International Classification of Diseases. In contrast, nonlicensed practitioners, such as optimal performance consultants may use neurofeedback training to enhance the client's quality of life or performance in a given field.[37–39] The Biofeedback Certification International Alliance (BCIA) certifies individuals who meet education and training standards in biofeedback and neurofeedback. BCIA certification, however, is not a substitute for a state-issued license or other professional credential.

Clinical Guidelines for Neurofeedback

When is it appropriate to refer a patient to a neurofeedback consultant? An obvious instance is if the patient has nonresponse or insufficient response to standard treatments and/or intolerance of medication side effects. Positive indicators for a trial of neurofeedback include the following: deficits in cognition, attention problems with or without hyperactivity, fatigue, sleep disturbance, mood dysregulation, chronic pain or seizures, or other disorders with underlying central nervous system dysregulation. Neurofeedback can be used as a stand-alone or adjunctive treatment. It has been used successfully as an adjunct to medication, psychotherapy, cognitive behavioral therapy, and Alcoholics Anonymous support for relapse prevention in the treatment of substance abusers.[40,41]

APPENDIX: REFERENCES

The complete reference list is online at http://www.psych.theclinics.com/dx.doi.org/10.1016/j.psc.2013.01.005.

KEY REFERENCES

2. Larsen S. The neurofeedback solution. Rochester (VT): Healing Arts Press; 2012.
3. Sherlin L, Arns M, Lubar J, et al. Neurofeedback and basic learning theory: implications for research and practice. J Neurother 2011;15(4):292–304.
4. Thomas JL. Neurofeedback: a new modality for treating brain problems. Archives of Medical Psychology 2012;3(1). Available at: http://www.amphome.org/archives/ArchivesMay2012. Accessed November 22, 2012.
16. Gevensleben H, Holl B, Albrecht B, et al. Is neurofeedback an efficacious treatment for ADHD? A randomised controlled clinical trial. J Child Psychol Psychiatry 2009;50(7):780–9.
17. Wyrwicka W, Sterman MB. Instrumental conditioning of sensorimotor cortex EEG spindles in the waking cat. Physiol Behav 1968;3(5):703–7.
19. Lubar JF, Lubar JO. Neurofeedback assessment and treatment for attention deficit/hyperactivity disorders (ADD/HD). In: Evans J, Abarbanel A, editors. Introduction to quantitative EEG and Neurotherapy. Academic Press; 1999. p. 103–43.
20. Sherlin L, Arns M, Lubar JF, et al. A position paper on neurofeedback for the treatment of ADHD. J Neurother 2010;14(2):66–78. Available at: http://dx.doi.org/10.1080/10874201003773880.
21. Arns M, de Ridder S, Strehl U, et al. Efficacy of neurofeedback treatment in ADHD: the effects on inattention, impulsivity and hyperactivity: a meta-analysis. Clin EEG Neurosci 2009;40(3):180–9.
28. Larsen S. The healing power of neurofeedback. Rochester (VT): Healing Arts Press; 2006.
32. Hammond DC, Kirk L. First, do no harm: adverse effects and the need for practice standards in neurofeedback. J Neurother 2008;12(1):79–88. http://dx.doi.org/10.1080/10874200802219947.

Cranial Electrotherapy Stimulation for Treatment of Anxiety, Depression, and Insomnia

Daniel L. Kirsch, PhD[a],*, Francine Nichols, RN, PhD[b]

KEYWORDS

- Cranial electrotherapy stimulation • CES • Anxiety • Depression • Insomnia

KEY POINTS

- Cranial electrotherapy stimulation (CES) is a US Food and Drug Administration–approved, prescriptive, noninvasive electromedical treatment that has been shown to decrease anxiety, insomnia, and depression significantly.
- Side effects from CES are mild and self-limiting (<1%); these include vertigo, skin irritation at electrode sites, and headaches.
- A functional magnetic resonance imaging study showed that CES causes cortical deactivation, producing changes similar to those produced by anxiolytic medications. Electroencephalographic studies show that CES increases alpha activity (increased relaxation), decreases delta activity (reduced fatigue), and decreased beta activity (decreased ruminative thoughts).
- Neurotransmitter studies revealed that CES increased blood plasma levels of β endorphin, adrenocorticotrophic hormone, serotonin, melatonin, norepinephrine, and cholinesterase. CES also decreased serum cortisol levels.
- CES treatments are cumulative; however, most patients show at least some improvement after the first treatment. Depression can take up to 3 weeks for initial response. Insomnia varies widely with some individuals having improved sleep immediately and others not having improved sleep until 2 months into treatment.
- A trial treatment in the office or clinic can identify those individuals who readily respond to CES treatment. CES can also be used during psychotherapy sessions and with medications, hypnosis, and biofeedback to decrease patient anxiety.
- CES is cost-effective compared with drugs and other devices used in psychiatry. It is easy to use in both clinical and home settings.

Conflict of Interest: D.K. is Chairman of Electromedical Products International, Inc; F.N. is Research Consultant for Electromedical Products International, Inc.
[a] The American Institute of Stress, 9112 Camp Bowie West Boulevard #228, Fort Worth, TX 76116, USA; [b] Georgetown University, Washington, DC, USA
* Corresponding author. 2201 Garrett Morris Parkway, Mineral Wells, TX 76067.
E-mail address: dkirsch@stress.org

INTRODUCTION

Cranial electrotherapy stimulation (CES) uses medical devices about the size of a cell phone that send a pulsed, weak electrical current (<4 mA) to the brain via electrodes placed on the ear lobes, maxilla-occipital junction, mastoid processes, or temples. CES was first cleared for interstate marketing and export by the US Food and Drug Administration for the treatment of anxiety, depression, and insomnia in 1979 and its use in clinical practice has steadily increased over time. The primary treatments used today for anxiety, depression, and insomnia are pharmaceuticals and psychotherapy. Both approaches have limitations in terms of effectiveness, side effects, costs, or time required. During the last decade, an increasing number of psychiatrists are integrating CES treatments into their clinical practice because it is noninvasive, has few side effects (1% or less), and treats anxiety, depression, and insomnia simultaneously. However, many clinicians are still unfamiliar with the considerable scientific evidence demonstrating the efficacy of some CES devices. This article summarizes neurophysiologic effects and the clinical research on CES as well as methods for integrating CES into the treatment of anxiety, depression, and insomnia.

NEUROPHYSIOLOGIC EFFECTS AND RESEARCH STUDIES

The brain functions electrochemically and can be readily modulated by electrical intervention. Research conducted at the Biomedical Engineering Program of the University of Texas at Austin indicated that from 1 mA of current, about 5 μA/cm^2 of CES reaches the thalamic area at a radius of 13.30 mm and may facilitate the release of neurotransmitters, which in turn could cause physiologic effects such as relaxation.[1] CES is believed to affect the subcortical brain structures known to regulate emotions, such as the reticular activating system, thalamus, and hypothalamus, as well as the limbic system. CES may stimulate regions that regulate pain messages, neurotransmitter function, and hormone production via the hypothalamic-pituitary axis.[2] CES treatments induce significant changes in the electroencephalogram, increasing alpha (8–12 Hz) relative power and decreasing relative power in the delta (0–3.5 Hz) and beta (12.5–30 Hz) frequencies.[3] Increased alpha correlates with improved relaxation and increased mental alertness or clarity. Decreased delta waves indicate a reduction in fatigue. Beta-wave reductions between 20 and 30 Hz correlate with decreases in anxiety, ruminative thoughts, and obsessive/compulsive-like behaviors.

Low-resolution electromagnetic tomography and functional magnetic resonance imaging studies showed that CES reached all cortical and subcortical areas of the brain, producing changes similar to those induced by anxiolytic medications.[4,5] Many symptoms seen in psychiatric conditions, such as anxiety, insomnia, and attention deficit disorders, are thought to be exacerbated by excess cortical activation.[6,7] A recent functional magnetic resonance imaging study showed that CES causes cortical brain deactivation in the midline frontal and parietal regions of the brain after one 20-minute treatment.[4]

CES treatments have been found to induce changes in neurohormones and neurotransmitters that have been implicated in psychiatric disorders: substantial increases in beta endorphins, adrenocorticotrophic hormone, and serotonin; moderate increases in melatonin and norepinephrine, modest or unquantified increases in cholinesterase, gamma-aminobutyric acid, and dehydroepiandrosterone, and moderate reductions in cortisol.[8,9] **Table 1** shows some of the chemical changes associated with use of the LISS CES device.

Table 1
Mean changes in neurochemicals in blood plasma after one 20-minute CES session

Neurochemical	Change	Implications
Beta endorphin	↑ 98%	Decreases pain
Adrenocorticotrophic hormone	↑ 75%	Promotes homeostasis
Serotonin (5HT)	↑ 50%	Improves mood Increases pain tolerance Decreases insomnia
Melatonin	↑ 25%	Induces sleep
Norepinephrine	↑ 24%	Increases pleasure Increases arousal
Cortisol	↓ 18%	Reduces stress response
Cholinesterase	↑ 8%	Increases relaxation
gamma-Aminobutyric acid	↑[a]	Decreases spasticity
Dehydroepiandrosterone	↑[a]	Improves immune system functioning

[a] Percentage increase not stated in source.

Cranial Electrotherapy Stimulation for Anxiety, Depression, Insomnia

There is a wealth of data on CES from more than 40 years of research. In 3 randomized, double-blind, sham-controlled studies and 1 investigator-blind study with a control group that included 227 subjects, the active CES groups had significantly lower scores on anxiety outcome measures than the sham or control groups.[10–13] Effect sizes ranged from $d = -0.60$ (moderate) to $d = -0.88$ (high). Effect sizes from 2 open clinical trials (N = 208) investigating the efficacy of CES for anxiety were also robust at $d = -0.75$ (moderate) and $d = -1.52$ (very high) on the Four-dimensional Anxiety and Depression Scale and the Hamilton Anxiety Rating Scale (HARS), respectively.[14,15] CES was also shown to decrease depression[14,16] and insomnia significantly.[17,18] These studies used the Alpha-Stim (Electromedical Products International, Inc, Mineral Wells, Texas) brand of CES device with reliable and valid outcome measurement scales. A limitation of these CES randomized controlled trials (RCT) is that they were small with the number of subjects ranging from 33 to 74. These studies need to be replicated with a larger number of subjects. Three studies[11–13] used a rigorous double-blind, sham-controlled RCT design, whereas the remaining studies cited were RCTs or open-label studies. Additional, ongoing double-blind, sham-controlled RCTs with larger numbers of subjects, funded by the National Institutes of Health, Department of Defense, and Veterans Administration, will strengthen the evidence for CES treatments.

Cranial Electrotherapy Stimulation for Assaultive Behavior

Preliminary research on the use of CES in psychiatric populations is extending to assaultive behaviors. Forty-eight chronically aggressive neuropsychiatric patients were treated for at least 2 to 3 months with CES at North Texas State Hospital at Vernon, a maximum security psychiatric hospital.[19]

- The patients, ages 18 to 62, had been hospitalized from a few months to more than 20 years and included many of the most resistant patients in the maximum security unit.
- The patients remained on their antipsychotic and mood stabilizing medications during CES.

- Every patient had multiple comorbidities: 45 of the 48 carried psychotic diagnoses; mental retardation was present in 31, and central nervous system trauma was etiologic in 6. Well-controlled seizure disorders were noted in 18.
- Some form of personality disorder was diagnosed in almost all cases, but only 3 were diagnosed primarily with antisocial personality disorder.
- Two patients had Huntington chorea, and 2 others had pervasive developmental disorder with psychosis.
- One patient met criteria for intermittent explosive disorder.
- Psychotic diagnoses included schizoaffective disorder, 12 (all manic); disorganized schizophrenia, 8; paranoid schizophrenia, 7; undifferentiated schizophrenia, 5; and bipolar disorder (manic), 2.
- Of the 48, 41 had been declared manifestly dangerous.
- The remaining 7 patients had been found incompetent to stand trial on felony charges involving bodily injury.

Forty of the 48 (83%) responded positively to CES. In the 3 months before CES, the group committed 1301 acts of aggression. During the 3 months of active CES treatment, there were 767 acts of aggression, a decline of 41% ($P<.001$). Seclusions declined 40% ($P = .05$) from 199 to 120, and the number of times patients required restraint decreased 40% ($P<.001$) from 446 to 268. Frequency of PRN medication declined 42% ($P<.01$) from 648 times over 3 months pretreatment to 377 times during 3 months of active treatment. The decrease of 271 PRN medication doses in 3 months resulted in a savings of more than $12,000 for these medication expenses alone. Overall, 32 of the 48 patients were able to be discharged from the hospital, and none returned for at least 2 years, as of the presentation by Childs at the American Psychiatric Association annual conference in 2007. Five of the 6 central nervous system trauma cases improved. Among the 7 patients previously incompetent to stand trial, 6 who responded to CES were subsequently found competent and have been returned to the courts for judicial processing. Two other patients, one of whom was primarily antisocial, and the other with pronounced antisocial traits, were nonresponders to CES.

CLINICAL CONSIDERATIONS AND GUIDELINES

To integrate CES into the practice of psychiatry for the treatment of anxiety, posttraumatic stress disorder, depression, and insomnia, the authors recommend a trial series of treatments in a clinic or office to evaluate responses in each individual. After the initial trial, patients can be prescribed a CES device to use at home, giving them increased control over the management of their symptoms. In addition to a regular 20- to 60-minute treatment daily or every other day, patients can add treatments as needed. Some clinicians find it useful to set up a CES lounge where patients can come in for treatments whenever they feel stressed.

Cranial Electrotherapy Stimulation During Psychotherapy Sessions

CES may also be used during psychotherapy sessions. Using CES during a therapy session decreases anxiety and usually improves the patient's ability to share problems, concerns, and worries with the therapist, as well as to respond to the therapist's questions more effectively. Anecdotal reports from psychiatrists and other mental health professionals on the use of CES during therapy are consistently enthusiastic. CES induces a prehypnotic relaxed state of mind and body that is complementary with many other interventions.

Concurrent Pharmacotherapy

CES can be used with pharmacologic therapy without concern about potential medication interactions. However, it is important to inform the patient that CES may decrease the need for medication. As the patient improves, both the psychiatrist and the patient should be alert for symptoms that may indicate a need for a dosage adjustment.[20]

Self-directed Home Treatment

Most individuals are capable of doing self-directed CES therapy at home. Treatments may need to be performed daily during the first 1 to 3 or 4 weeks and then 2 to 3 times per week during a maintenance phase. The individual can also use CES as often as needed, as there are no side effects from extended use, which is especially beneficial for those individuals diagnosed with posttraumatic stress disorder and those who experience panic attacks.

EVALUATING IMMEDIATE AND LONG-TERM EFFECTS

Feelings experienced during a CES treatment are shown in **Fig. 1**. If the patient feels heavy, groggy, or euphoric at the end of the allotted time, it is important to continue the treatment session until the patient feels "light." At the end of a CES session, most patients will feel more relaxed, yet alert, and have an increased sense of well-being.

Evaluating a single 20- to 40-minute trial of CES in a clinic or office will help identify those individuals who most readily respond to CES. However, CES effects are cumulative so those who do not respond initially may benefit when given daily treatments (20–60 minutes) for 1 month or longer.[21]

A psychiatrist who would like to document treatment progress in CES patients may chose to use the HARS, Hamilton Depression Rating Scale 17, and/or the Pittsburgh Sleep Quality Index, all of which have proven useful in evaluating CES outcomes. The

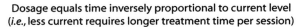

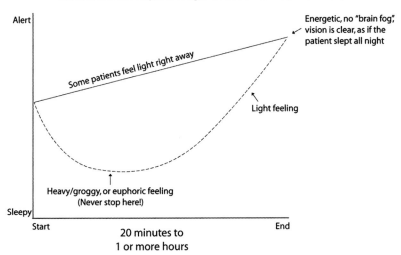

Fig. 1. Feelings experienced during CES treatment stages.

HARS should be administered before and immediately after the first treatment and after 3 weeks and 6 weeks of daily use. For depression and insomnia, which typically respond more slowly, patients should be tested before, but not immediately after, the first treatment. Measurements at 3 weeks and 6 weeks provide useful assessments of patient progress.

CONTRAINDICATIONS, PRECAUTIONS, AND ADVERSE EFFECTS OF CRANIAL ELECTROTHERAPY STIMULATION

There are no known contraindications to the use of CES. The only precaution is regarding use during pregnancy. A study of potential teratogenic effects from CES was conducted on 844 Spraque-Dawley fetal rats.[22] The treated rats were divided into 3 groups and given CES 1 hour daily throughout their pregnancy at either 10, 100, or 1000 Hz, while the parameters of 1 V, 0.125 mA, at a 0.22-microseconds pulse width remained constant. On day 18 of pregnancy, the dams were killed and cesarean section was performed immediately. After thorough external examination, autopsies evaluated the palate, heart, major vessels, lungs, liver, kidneys, ureters, and bladder. Examinations under light microscopy revealed no neural tube defects, limb reduction deformities, or anterior abdominal wall abnormalities in the controls or in any of the treatment groups. Skeletal surveys of the fetal rats found no vertebral column, rib, or long bone deformities. Comparison between groups revealed more pregnancy resorptions and fewer offspring in all treatment groups compared with the control group, with the difference only reaching significance in the 1000-Hz treatment group. Average fetal weights were inversely proportional to frequency and were significantly different among groups. Fetal brain weight followed a similar pattern of reduction, except that weights were not significantly different between the medium and highest frequency treatment groups.

In their discussion, the researchers stated that, whereas the incidence of congenital anomalies was zero, the reason pregnancy resorptions were increased may be due to the CES-treated rats being more complacent. Their behavior resembled the calming effects of CES in humans. The treated rats were not as active as the control rats. Accordingly, it is possible that food intake was lowered in the treatment group, a reasonable implication given the reduction in fetal weights. They concluded that CES may be embryolethal in the very early stages of pregnancy in the rat and might cause some miscarriages, especially at 1000 Hz, but there is no evidence of fetotoxic effects. The relevance of these findings to humans is unknown.

Adverse effects of CES in humans occur in less than 1% of cases and they are usually mild and self-limiting. These adverse effects include vertigo, skin irritation at electrode sites, and headaches. Headaches and vertigo are usually associated with the current being set too high for the individual. These effects resolve when the current is reduced or within minutes to hours following treatment. Irritation at the electrode site can be avoided by moving electrodes around slightly during treatments. No serious adverse effect has ever been reported from using CES.[23]

SUMMARY

CES can improve the safety and efficacy of treatment of anxiety, insomnia, and depression. When prescribed for home use, patients are empowered to regulate their own moods and to overcome their sleep problems, thus enhancing patient outcomes. Compared with other neuerostimulation techniques for brain repair, CES is noninvasive and less expensive and can be used safely and conveniently by patients at home. It is useful as an adjunct to medication or psychotherapy or as a stand-alone treatment. Historically CES has been used as a last resort when medications and other interventions fail or are not well tolerated. With an increase in the evidence base for positive outcomes, more physicians are recognizing CES as a first-line or adjunctive treatment.

REFERENCES

1. Ferdjallah M, Bostick FX, Barr RE. Potential and current density distributions of cranial electrotherapy stimulation (CES) in a four concentric-spheres model. IEEE Trans Biomed Eng 1996;43:939–43.
2. Kirsch DL. Cranial electrotherapy stimulation for the treatment of anxiety, depression, insomnia and other conditions. Insert: Giordano, James. Illustrating how CES works. Nat Med 2006;23:118–20.
3. Kennerly R. QEEG analysis of cranial electrotherapy: a pilot study. J Neurother 2004;8:112–3.
4. Feusner JD, Madsen S, Moody TD, et al. Effects of cranial electrotherapy stimulation on resting state brain activity. Brain Behav 2012;2(3):211–20.
5. Kennerly RC. Changes in quantitative EEG and low resolution tomography following cranial electrotherapy stimulation. Ph.D. Dissertation, the University of North Texas. 529 pp, 81 tables, 233 figures, 171 references, 2006.
6. Yassa MA, Hazlett RL, Stark CE, et al. Functional MRI of the amygdala and bed nucleus of the stria terminalis during conditions of uncertainty in generalized anxiety disorder. J Psychiatr Res 2012;46:1045–52.
7. Bonnet MH, Arand DL. Hyperarousal and insomnia: state of the science. Sleep Med Rev 2010;14:9–15.
8. Shealy CN, Cady RK, Culver-Veehoff D, et al. Cerebrospinal fluid and plasma neurochemicals: response to cranial electrical stimulation. J Neuro Orthop Med Surg 1998;18:94–7.
9. Liss S, Liss B. Physiological and therapeutic effects of high frequency electrical pulses. Integr Physiol Behav Sci 1996;31:88–96.
10. Kim HJ, Kim WY, Lee YS, et al. The effect of cranial electrotherapy stimulation on preoperative anxiety and hemodynamic responses. Korean J Anesthesiol 2008;55:657–61.
11. Cork RC, Wood PM, Norbert C, et al. The effect of cranial electrotherapy stimulation (CES) on pain associated with fibromyalgia. Internet J Anesthesiol 2004;8:1–7.
12. Lichtbroun AS. The treatment of fibromyalgia with cranial electrotherapy stimulation. J Clin Rheumatol 2001;7:72–8.
13. Winick RL. Cranial electrotherapy stimulation (CES): a safe and effective low cost means of anxiety control in a dental practice. Gen Dent 1999;47:50–5.
14. Bystritsky A, Kerwin L, Feusner JD. A pilot study of cranial electrotherapy stimulation for generalized anxiety disorder. J Clin Psychiatry 2008;69:412–7.
15. Overcash SJ. Cranial electrotherapy stimulation in patients suffering from acute anxiety disorders. American J Electromed 1999;16:49–51.
16. Kirsch DL, Gilula M. Cranial electrotherapy stimulation in the treatment of depression – part 2. Pract Pain Manag 2007;7:32–40.
17. Taylor AG, Anderson JG, Riedel SL, et al. Cranial electrical stimulation improves symptoms and functional status in individuals with fibromyalgia. Pain Manag Nurs, in press.
18. Kirsch DL, Gilula MF. CES in the treatment of insomnia: a review and meta-analysis. Pract Pain Manag 2007;7:30–43.

19. Childs A, Price L. Cranial electrotherapy stimulation reduces aggression in violent neuropsychiatric patients. Prim Psychiatr 2007;14:50–6.
20. Stanley TH, Cazalaa JA. Transcutaneous cranial electrical stimulation decreases narcotic requirements during neurolept anesthesia and operation in man. Anesth Analg 1982;61:863–6.
21. Holubec JT. Cumulative response from cranial electrotherapy stimulation (CES) for chronic pain. Pract Pain Manag 2009;9:80–3.
22. Little B, Patterson MA. Embryofetal effects of neuroelectric therapy (NET). Electromagnetic Biology and Medicine 1996;15(1):1–8.
23. Electromedical Products International, Inc, CES safety data submitted to FDA, February 10, 2012. Available at: http://www.alpha-stim.com/wp-content/uploads/EPIs-fda-presentation.pdf. Accessed November 2, 2012.

Testosterone and Mood in Aging Men

Stuart N. Seidman, MD[a,c,*], Mark Weiser, MD[b,c]

KEYWORDS

- Testosterone • Partial androgen deficiency of aging male
- Hypothalamic-pituitary-gonadal axis • Depression

KEY POINTS

- Testosterone level is reduced with age.
- Partial androgen deficiency of the aging male (PADAM) is thought to be responsible for a variety of age-associated conditions, such as reduced muscle and bone mass, frailty, sexual dysfunction, and depression.
- Testosterone deficiency is most consistently associated with sexual dysfunction and fatigue, and these are reversed by testosterone replacement.
- There is only limited evidence of a link between hypothalamic-pituitary-gonadal axis hypo-functioning and depressive illness.
- Exogenous testosterone has not been consistently shown to be effective for major depressive disorder in either hypogonadal or eugonadal men; some evidence supports a mood-enhancing effect in men with late-onset dysthymia (which may be considered a PADAM manifestation in some men).

INTRODUCTION

Male hypothalamic-pituitary-gonadal (HPG) axis function declines progressively after age 40 years, and about one-fourth of middle-aged and older men have testosterone levels below the threshold values used to define testosterone deficiency in younger men.[1,2] Of these, less than half exhibit apparent sequelae of low testosterone levels, meeting the definition of hypogonadism.[1,2] Mild testosterone deficiency in men can be considered physiologic (ie, a para-aging phenomenon) or pathologic (ie, a deficit state). Indeed, whether the age-dependent decline in testosterone levels truly causes health problems in men is being debated vigorously.[3–7] It has been suggested that age-associated testosterone deficiency, termed partial androgen deficiency of the aging male (PADAM), is responsible for many of the typical signs of male aging, such as sexual dysfunction, decreased lean body mass, osteoporosis, and increased

a West End Medical Associates, 617 West End Avenue, New York, NY 10024, USA; b Department of Psychiatry, Sackler Faculty of Medicine, Tel Aviv University, Ramat Aviv 69978, Israel; c Department of Psychiatry, Sheba Medical Center, Tel-Hashomer 52621, Israel
* Corresponding author.
E-mail address: stuart.seidman@yahoo.com

Psychiatr Clin N Am 36 (2013) 177–182
http://dx.doi.org/10.1016/j.psc.2013.01.007
0193-953X/13/$ – see front matter © 2013 Elsevier Inc. All rights reserved.

visceral fat, as well as for neuropsychiatric problems such as fatigue, depression, and irritability.[7–12] Furthermore, it is claimed that the application of a testosterone replacement strategy for older men with low or low to normal testosterone levels will reverse such presumed sequelae.[13]

In contrast to PADAM "enthusiasts," other investigators have shown that for many, hypogonadism is not a stable health state (eg, in a 15-year longitudinal follow-up of a large population-based sample of men, the majority of those with low testosterone level remit to normal levels in later years[4]); aside from sexual dysfunction and fatigue,[12,14] hormone levels do not correlate with most of the presumed hypogonadal symptoms[8,9,15] although age and illness do[9,10]; and testosterone replacement in elderly men is mostly ineffective in reversing most of these signs and symptoms.[6,10] Finally, the limited data that exist regarding mood effects of endogenous and exogenous testosterone in this population are inconsistent, but broadly unsupportive of a role in major depression or its treatment.[7,16] There is some evidence that testosterone may play a more pivotal role in later-onset, low-grade depressive syndromes, such as dysthymia.[17,18]

LATE-ONSET MALE HYPOGONADISM

It is controversial whether age should be considered the primary variable linked to "age-related" testosterone decline because there are many influences on HPG-axis functioning, including genetic factors, chronic diseases, medications, obesity, and lifestyle factors.[11] Indeed, poor health is a better predictor than age of decline in testosterone level.[7] Although many men with low testosterone levels are asymptomatic, others may have a partial decline in testosterone associated with various clinical symptoms.[9,12] Of note, there appear to be different thresholds for different hypogonadal symptoms: loss of vigor and libido (<430 ng/dL), obesity (<346 ng/dL), disturbed sleep, depression, poor concentration (<288 ng/dL), and hot flushes (<230 ng/dL).[7] There is also variability in the time course of symptom reversal following testosterone replacement.[19] Based on the linkage of symptoms with androgenic actions, it remains unclear whether PADAM—an age-related hypogonadal syndrome characterized by sexual, somatic, and behavioral symptoms, with insidious onset and slow progression—is a true clinical entity distinguishable from age-related and health-related changes and frailty.

MALE HPG AXIS AND DEPRESSION
Exogenous Testosterone Administration in Depressed Men

Reports from the older psychiatric literature (1935–1960) on the antidepressant effects of testosterone suggested that a substantial number of "depressed" men responded immediately and dramatically to hormone replacement therapy and subsequently relapsed when treatment was discontinued.[20] However, standardized, syndromal, psychiatric diagnoses were not used in these studies, baseline testosterone levels were not assessed, and there was no control group. Anecdotal reports over the past 2 decades have suggested that in some hypogonadal men, comorbid major depressive disorder (MDD) remits with testosterone replacement or testosterone augmentation of a partially effective antidepressant,[21] and that for men infected by the human immunodeficiency virus, testosterone replacement is associated with improved mood, libido, and energy.[22] Yet systematic study has not supported the initial enthusiasm for testosterone as an antidepressant.

In a double-blind, randomized clinical trial of testosterone replacement versus placebo in 30 men with MDD and hypogonadism, Seidman and colleagues[23] found testosterone replacement to be indistinguishable from placebo in antidepressant efficacy:

- 38% responded to testosterone
- 41% responded to placebo

An influential placebo-controlled trial of testosterone replacement as an augmentation to serotonergic antidepressant partial response suggested that this strategy might be more promising.[24] However, this was not supported by double-blind, placebo-controlled follow-up studies on antidepressant augmentation[25,26] or by a larger replication of the original study.[27]

Among older dysthymic men with low testosterone levels, 2 small placebo-controlled trials demonstrated a mood-enhancing effect of testosterone replacement.[17,18] Such data support the hypothesis that dysthymia is the psychiatric manifestation of PADAM, and that testosterone replacement is an effective treatment, but more systematic study is warranted before such conclusions can be made. At present, available data do not suggest the use of exogenous testosterone in the treatment of depression in PADAM, and clinical guidelines for hypogonadal men stress that testosterone replacement therapy for depression is not supported.[7,28]

Exogenous Testosterone: Clinical Considerations

Exogenous testosterone, even at supraphysiologic doses, rarely produces side effects, although there is a remote risk of developing gynecomastia (breast tenderness and breast enlargement), truncal acne (particularly for those with a history of acne), hair loss or hair growth, and/or induction or worsening of obstructive sleep apnea.[29] Because there is always a modest increase in hematocrit, complete blood count should be checked pretreatment and followed.[30] Via the negative feedback mechanism, exogenous testosterone suppresses luteinizing hormone and follicle-stimulating hormone, which leads to reduced testicular sperm production and, consequently, reduced testicular volume. Formulation-specific adverse effects include skin reactions at application site for transdermal patches, skin irritation from transdermal gel, pain at injection site, excessive erythrocytosis (especially in older patients), and coughing episodes immediately after the intramuscular injection of testosterone enanthate, cypionate, or undecanoate.[7]

The primary concern regarding potential adverse effects of testosterone treatment is related to the prostate gland. Androgens play a permissive role in the growth of prostate cancer and benign prostate hyperplasia (BPH); however, there are no data to indicate that testosterone administration can lead to the progression of preclinical prostate cancer or to worsening BPH.[7,29,31] Prostate cancer is an absolute contraindication to treatment with exogenous testosterone, and should be excluded in all men age 50 years and older (or older than 40 if there is a positive family history of prostate cancer) via pretreatment prostate-specific antigen and digital rectal examination of the prostate.[31,32] Finally, although most data support an improvement in cardiovascular health with testosterone replacement,[7] the TOM (Testosterone in Older Men with Sarcopenia) study, in which 209 elderly hypogonadal men were randomized to testosterone gel or placebo, needed to be stopped because of a significant increase in nonfatal cardiovascular adverse events (affecting 23 men in the testosterone group and 5 in the placebo group).[33] Although unique aspects of the trial have been used to explain this unexpected result, the experience has given pause to the testosterone replacement enthusiasts and has encouraged greater precision in defining indications for testosterone replacement in elderly men.

SUMMARY

In contrast to extensive menopause research, there is no parallel characterization of the psychophysiology of age-related male hypogonadism, despite potential implications for the treatment of psychiatric and sexual problems in this population. Nonetheless, the past decade has seen significant market growth in testosterone therapies for men 40 years and older, with most presumed indications lacking a firm scientific basis.

It is possible that an age-related hypogonadal syndrome, PADAM, is relevant to some men, and may include neuropsychiatric (including depressive) symptoms related to biological and psychosocial changes, and an individual's adaptation to such changes.[34] Although systematic study of the efficacy of exogenous testosterone in the treatment of depression in elderly hypogonadal men has been inconclusive, the great variability of the results suggests that in individual cases testosterone supplementation may be a useful adjunctive therapy in depressed (particularly dysthymic) hypogonadal men[17,18] for sexual dysfunction (including sexual dysfunction caused by antidepressant use[35]) and for frailty.[7,36]

REFERENCES

1. Araujo AB, Esche GR, Kupelian V, et al. Prevalence of symptomatic androgen deficiency in men. J Clin Endocrinol Metab 2007;92:4241–7.
2. Liu CC, Wu WJ, Lee YC, et al. The prevalence of and risk factors for androgen deficiency in aging Taiwanese men. J Sex Med 2009;6:936–46.
3. Seidman SN. Androgens and the aging male. Psychopharmacol Bull 2007;40:205–18.
4. Travison TG, Shackelton R, Araujo AB, et al. The natural history of symptomatic androgen deficiency in men: onset, progression, and spontaneous remission. J Am Geriatr Soc 2008;56:831–9.
5. Wang C, Nieschlag E, Swerdloff R, et al. Investigation, treatment, and monitoring of late-onset hypogonadism in males: ISA, ISSAM, EAU, EAA, and ASA recommendations. J Androl 2009;30:1–9.
6. Makinen JI, Huhtaniemi I. Androgen replacement therapy in late-onset hypogonadism: current concepts and controversies—a mini-review. Gerontology 2011;57:193–202.
7. Buvat J, Maggi M, Guay A, et al. Testosterone deficiency in men: systematic review and standard operating procedures for diagnosis and treatment. J Sex Med 2013;10(1):245–84.
8. Spetz AC, Palmefors L, Skobe RS, et al. Testosterone correlated to symptoms of partial androgen deficiency in aging men (PADAM) in an elderly Swedish population. Menopause 2007;14:999–1005.
9. Chueh KS, Huang SP, Lee YC, et al. The comparison of the aging male symptoms (AMS) scale and androgen deficiency in the aging male (ADAM) questionnaire to detect androgen deficiency in middle-aged men. J Androl 2012;33:817–23.
10. Emmelot-Vonk MH, Verhaar HJ, Nakhai-Pour HR, et al. Low testosterone concentrations and the symptoms of testosterone deficiency according to the androgen deficiency in ageing males (ADAM) and ageing males' symptoms rating scale (AMS) questionnaires. Clin Endocrinol (Oxf) 2011;74:488–94.
11. Amore M, Innamorati M, Costi S, et al. Partial androgen deficiency, depression, and testosterone supplementation in aging men. Int J Endocrinol 2012;2012:280724.
12. Wu FC, Tajar A, Beynon JM, et al. Identification of late-onset hypogonadism in middle-aged and elderly men. N Engl J Med 2010;363:123–35.

13. Bassil N, Morley JE. Late-life onset hypogonadism: a review. Clin Geriatr Med 2010;26:197–222.

14. Rosen RC, Araujo AB, Connor MK, et al. The NERI Hypogonadism Screener: psychometric validation in male patients and controls. Clin Endocrinol (Oxf) 2011;74:248–56.

15. McKinlay JB, Longcope C, Gray A. The questionable physiologic and epidemiologic basis for a male climacteric syndrome: preliminary results from the Massachusetts Male Aging Study. Maturitas 1989;11:103–15.

16. Amiaz R, Seidman SN. Testosterone and depression in men. Curr Opin Endocrinol Diabetes Obes 2008;15:278–83.

17. Seidman SN, Orr G, Raviv G, et al. Effects of testosterone replacement in middle-aged men with dysthymia: a randomized, placebo-controlled clinical trial. J Clin Psychopharmacol 2009;29:216–21.

18. Shores MM, Kivlahan DR, Sadak TI, et al. A randomized, double-blind, placebo-controlled study of testosterone treatment in hypogonadal older men with subthreshold depression (dysthymia or minor depression). J Clin Psychiatry 2009;70:1009–16.

19. Jockenhovel F, Minnemann T, Schubert M, et al. Timetable of effects of testosterone administration to hypogonadal men on variables of sex and mood. Aging Male 2009;12:113–8.

20. Seidman SN, Walsh BT. Testosterone and depression in aging men. Am J Geriatr Psychiatry 1999;7:18–33.

21. Seidman SN, Rabkin JG. Testosterone replacement therapy for hypogonadal men with SSRI-refractory depression. J Affect Disord 1998;48:157–61.

22. Rabkin JG, Wagner GJ, McElhiney MC, et al. Testosterone versus fluoxetine for depression and fatigue in HIV/AIDS: a placebo-controlled trial. J Clin Psychopharmacol 2004;24:379–85.

23. Seidman SN, Spatz E, Rizzo C, et al. Testosterone replacement therapy for hypogonadal men with major depressive disorder: a randomized, placebo-controlled clinical trial. J Clin Psychiatry 2001;62:406–12.

24. Pope HG, Cohane GH, Kanayama G, et al. Testosterone gel supplementation for men with refractory depression: a randomized, placebo-controlled trial. Am J Psychiatry 2003;160:105–11.

25. Seidman SN, Miyazaki M, Roose SP. Intramuscular testosterone supplementation to selective serotonin reuptake inhibitor in treatment-resistant depressed men: randomized placebo-controlled clinical trial. J Clin Psychopharmacol 2005;25:584–8.

26. Orengo CA, Fullerton L, Kunik ME. Safety and efficacy of testosterone gel 1% augmentation in depressed men with partial response to antidepressant therapy. J Geriatr Psychiatry Neurol 2005;18:20–4.

27. Pope HG Jr, Amiaz R, Brennan BP, et al. Parallel-group placebo-controlled trial of testosterone gel in men with major depressive disorder displaying an incomplete response to standard antidepressant treatment. J Clin Psychopharmacol 2010;30:126–34.

28. Bhasin S, Cunningham GR, Hayes FJ, et al. Testosterone therapy in men with androgen deficiency syndromes: an Endocrine Society clinical practice guideline. J Clin Endocrinol Metab 2010;95:2536–59.

29. Bhasin S, Basaria S. Diagnosis and treatment of hypogonadism in men. Best Pract Res Clin Endocrinol Metab 2011;25:251–70.

30. Bhasin S, Pencina M, Jasuja GK, et al. Reference ranges for testosterone in men generated using liquid chromatography tandem mass spectrometry in

a community-based sample of healthy nonobese young men in the Framingham Heart Study and applied to three geographically distinct cohorts. J Clin Endocrinol Metab 2011;96:2430–9.

31. Morgentaler A. Testosterone and prostate cancer: what are the risks for middle-aged men? Urol Clin North Am 2011;38:119–24.

32. Jannini EA, Gravina GL, Morgentaler A, et al. Is testosterone a friend or a foe of the prostate? J Sex Med 2011;8:946–55.

33. Basaria S, Coviello AD, Travison TG, et al. Adverse events associated with testosterone administration. N Engl J Med 2010;363:109–22.

34. Amore M. Partial androgen deficiency and neuropsychiatric symptoms in aging men. J Endocrinol Invest 2005;28:49–54.

35. Amiaz R, Pope HG Jr, Mahne T, et al. Testosterone gel replacement improves sexual function in depressed men taking serotonergic antidepressants: a randomized, placebo-controlled clinical trial. J Sex Marital Ther 2011;37:243–54.

36. Emmelot-Vonk MH, Verhaar ZH, Nakhai-Pour HA, et al. Effect of testosterone supplementation on functional mobility, cognition, and other parameters in older men: a randomized controlled trial. JAMA 2008;299:39–52.

Perinatal Depression and Anxiety
Beyond Psychopharmacology

Kelly Brogan, MD, ABIHM

KEYWORDS

- Postpartum depression • Mental disorders and pregnancy • Risk assessment
- Vitamin deficiency • Alternative therapies • Pregnancy nutrition

KEY POINTS

- The experience of pregnancy draws heavily on a woman's nutrient stores and involves fluctuations in hormone levels and immunologic parameters.
- Decision making in the treatment of mental disorders during pregnancy and lactation involves assessing relative risks of exposure to maternal illness and the potential adverse effects of nondrug treatments versus medications.
- A holistic approach endeavors to identify the systemic, root causes of illnesses and to provide patients with tools for self-care that extend beyond compliance with a prescription.

INTRODUCTION

Women of reproductive age represent a population whose treatment entails a complex web of risks and benefits. Between 10% and 18%[1] of women experience depression and anxiety during pregnancy and postpartum, when expectations are high for stability and wellness.

Risks associated with untreated maternal mental illness include poor self-care, substance abuse, medication exposures, preeclampsia, low birth weight, preterm birth, and neuropsychiatric sequelae in the child. Medication-associated concerns include neonatal adaptation syndrome, pulmonary hypertension, spontaneous abortion, low birth weight, and preterm labor. Although it is reassuring that, in more than 22,000 recorded exposures in the literature, no consistent findings indicate teratogenicity from antidepressants,[2] further prospective studies with longer follow-up and assessment are needed. A comprehensive approach to the care of a patient endeavors to identify root causes of illness (digestive, nutrient, hormonal, and fatty

Disclosures/Conflict of interest: None.
NYU/Bellevue Hospital Center, 280 Madison Avenue, Suite 702, New York, NY 10016, USA
E-mail address: drkellybrogan@kellybroganmd.com

Psychiatr Clin N Am 36 (2013) 183–188
http://dx.doi.org/10.1016/j.psc.2013.01.008
0193-953X/13/$ – see front matter © 2013 Elsevier Inc. All rights reserved.

acid imbalances) and to provide patients with tools for self-care that extend beyond compliance with a prescription.

COMPLEMENTS AND ALTERNATIVES TO PSYCHOPHARMACOLOGY DURING PREGNANCY

Women who are concerned about the use of traditional medications should be advised regarding the risks and benefits of treatment with bright light therapy, S-adenosylmethionine (SAMe), and cranial electrotherapy stimulation (CES), as well as supplementation with essential fatty acids, folate, and vitamin D.

Bright Light Therapy

Initially relegated to an evidence-based intervention for seasonal affective disorder, bright light therapy is used for treatment of pregnant patients. In an open study on antenatal major depression, 60 minutes of daily 10,000-lux light for 3 weeks resulted in a 49% improvement on the Hamilton Rating Scale for Depression. A 10-week, double-blind, randomized, placebo-controlled (DBRPC) trial of 7000 versus 500 lux showed an effect size of 0.43 for the 7000-lux group after 5 weeks, which is comparable with antidepressant treatment.[3] A typical regimen is 30 minutes of morning exposure to a UV-filtered, 10,000-lux lamp. Risks include headache and overactivation in patients with a history of bipolar disorder.

SAMe

SAMe is a naturally occurring methyl donor in the human body participating in essential metabolic pathways including the formation of neurotransmitters, methylation of phospholipids, glutathione synthesis, myelination, coenzyme q10, carnitine, creatine, and DNA transcription (see the Bottiglieri article in this issue). Dosing is usually 400 mg to 1600 mg/d and sometimes up to 2400 mg/d depending on severity and tolerance. No adverse effects were reported in 8 studies (total n = ~150) of SAMe in the treatment of women with cholestasis during pregnancy. In postpartum patients with subjective reports of depressive symptoms, SAMe in doses up to 1600 mg/d achieved a 75% reduction of symptoms in 30 days (50% in 10 days) relative to placebo.[4]

CES

Cranial electrical stimulators are patient-administered devices that are approved by the US Food and Drug Administration for treatment of anxiety, depression, and insomnia. The low-intensity alternating current transmitted across the skull for 20 minutes once or twice daily promotes alpha wave activity, and modulates neurotransmitters, endorphins, and cortisol (see the article in this issue by Kirsch and Nichols on Cranial Electrotherapy Stimulation).[5] There are no perinatal studies of the devices; however, given that the current used is less than that of a cell phone, adverse effects are unlikely. This device could become a first-line option for women because it is noninvasive and has a low side effect profile. The device requires a physician's prescription.

Fatty Acids

Cholesterol, phospholipids, free fatty acids, and triglycerides provide sources of energy storage, nuanced signaling systems as eicosanoid precursors, and provide structural support with a balance of rigidity and fluidity for membrane receptors, peptides, and channels. Linoleic acid and alpha-linolenic acid are essential acids (not endogenously synthesized) found in meats, nuts, and seeds like sunflower and flax. Humans are inefficient at converting these precursors into the highly unsaturated fats/eicosanoids such as the omega-6 fatty acids, dihomo-gamma-linolenic acid (DGLA) and arachidonic acid (AA) or the omega-3 fatty acid, eicosapentaenoic acid (EPA). As is conjectured in gestational diabetes, increased insulin and glucose levels may upregulate phospholipase A2, which cleaves fatty acids from phospholipids, disturbing membrane structure. The only means of assessing individual fatty acid needs is through erythrocyte analysis. Optimal dietary ratios range from 4:1 to 1:1, omega-6/omega-3, depending on the source consulted.

Epidemiologic data suggest that the prevalence of perinatal depression correlates inversely with fish consumption[6] and that low fish intake during pregnancy may raise the risk of treatment with an antidepressant for up to 1 year postpartum.[7] Three DBRPC trials have evaluated the relationship between omega-3 fatty acids and perinatal depression. Of the three studies, 2 have shown a significant benefit from omega-3 fatty acid in the treatment of depressive symptoms.[3] Recent meta-analyses support dosages of 3:2, EPA/DHA, 1 to 3 g total daily supplementation.[8,9]

There is a risk that chronic oversupplementation of omega-3 from flax and/or fish oil may impair production of omega-6 highly unsaturated fatty acids such as gamma-linolenic acid (GLA), DGLA, and AA (precursors to prostaglandin E1 [PGE1] and prostacyclin) and contribute to imbalance through competitive inhibition.[10–12] The effect of GLA administration can be simplistically attributed to production of the eicosanoid DGLA, which serves to regulate AA (promoting its retention in the membrane) through its conversion to PGE1. At least 3 randomized, placebo-controlled trials (RCTs) of evening primrose oil (0.5–2 mg) in premenstrual syndrome suggest that GLA is an effective intervention, possibly related to its potentiation of PGE1 and attenuation of prolactin sensitivity at the receptor site in the membrane.[13] A small DBRPC trial found evidence that, in healthy women supplemented with fish oil and evening primrose oil, fatty acid profiles showed increase in GLA, DGLA, and DHA levels without AA suppression.[14]

Folate

Folate (vitamin B_9), found in leafy greens, lentils, broccoli, and sunflower seeds, is an important cofactor in the synthesis of monoamines, reduction of homocysteine (with vitamin B_{12} as a cofactor), and slowing central nervous system breakdown of tryptophan through its conversion to l-methylfolate (see the Bottiglieri article in this issue). Maternal 5,10 methylene tetrahydrofolate reductase polymorphisms are associated with antenatal depression and may influence the fetal programming of serotonin transporter methylation and future functioning.[15] A recent study showed benefit, based on Edinburgh Postnatal Depression Scale scores, at 21 months postpartum for women with C677TT polymorphism who supplemented with folic acid during pregnancy.[16] Bypassing enzymatic conversion of folic acid to l-methylfolate with bioactive metabolite may be a potential treatment option.

Vitamin D

Vitamin D has myriad immune-modulating, bone supporting, and mood-modifying actions. A study of 178 pregnant African American women showed a relationship between low first-trimester 25-hydroxyvitamin D serum levels and second-trimester antenatal depression diagnosed by the Center for Epidemiologic Studies Depression Scale.[17] Supplementation to achieve serum 25-hydroxy vitamin D levels of more than 40 ng/mL often requires more than the recommended dose of 400 IU daily, and in some cases up to 4000 IU daily.[18] In an Amsterdam birth cohort, deficiency/insufficiency of vitamin D serum levels at 13 weeks' gestation was associated with significant depressive symptoms at 16 weeks' gestation.[19] Postpartum serum levels less than 32 ng/mL have correlated with increased incidence of depressive symptoms.[20]

EVALUATION OF POSTPARTUM MOOD AND ANXIETY SYMPTOMS
Nutrition

The evaluation of new-onset postpartum mood and anxiety includes a thorough assessment of nutritional risk factors (screening for serum levels of calcium, B_{12}/methylmalonic acid, folate, magnesium, and zinc). Although the fetus protects its needs, the mother's stores are often compromised. A study of pregnant American women found that most were consuming less than the recommended amounts of iron, zinc, calcium, magnesium, folate, and vitamins D and E.[21]

Immune Modulation

Immune modulation in the postpartum period contributes to a 10% incidence of postpartum thyroiditis with insomnia, anxiety, palpitations, irritability, and weight loss occurring 1 to 4 months postpartum, followed by hypothyroidism, which may present 4 to 8 months postpartum. Thyroid-secreting hormone (TSH) at delivery has been shown to be a predictor of postpartum depression at 6 months postpartum.[22] Of 31 inpatient women with a diagnosis of postpartum psychosis, 19% had detectable thyroid autoantibodies and 67% of these women developed thyroid dysfunction by 6 months, compared with 20% of controls.[23] Appropriate assessment entails screening for thyroid autoantibodies, levels of free hormones (T3 and T4), and TSH. For women with diagnosed hypothyroidism on T4 monotherapy, T3 may be an option as an augmentation before initiating antidepressant treatment. The rationale is based on limited central nervous system conversion of T4 to T3, a nutrient-dependent process impeded by increased cortisol.[24]

Inflammatory Cytokines

Specific inflammatory cytokines such as interleukin 1B have been identified as early warning indicators of depression developing at 1 month postpartum.[25] Generationally transferred alterations in microbial flora resulting from antibiotic medication or dietary exposures may account for intestinal dysbiosis and production of inflammatory cytokines by pathogenic bacteria and fungi. Two studies raised questions about the inflammatory role of processed foods such as gluten and dairy in the development of postpartum depression and psychosis, suggesting that plasma/cerebrospinal fluid morphinelike fragments derived from casein and gluten may have an association with maternal psychopathology[26] and possibly mental illness in the child.[27]

Neurotoxins

Other sources of oxidative stress include environmental exposures to chemicals that place a metabolic burden on the system. With 80,000 registered agents in the Toxic Substances Inventory, only 200 have been studied for human safety parameters. A case series supported by the Environmental Working Group examined umbilical cords and identified 287 toxic chemicals, 217 of which are known neurotoxins. Polybrominated diphenyl ether flame retardants, phthalates, and bisphenol A have been associated with adverse cognitive, endocrine, and motor outcomes in children,[28–30] and, although seemingly ubiquitous, represent a modifiable exposure. Women would be better able to reduce environmental risks if they were given information about potential adverse effects from untested chemicals in their cosmetics, pesticide-treated foods, water, air, and plastics.

SUMMARY

When a woman is planning a pregnancy, is pregnant, or postpartum, she may consult a mental health provider for expertise in the developing field of nonpharmacologic treatments. Complementary and alternative medicine improves the capacity of clinicians to individualize treatment options beyond prescription medication. Whether optimizing underlying nutritional factors associated with depression, such as folate, essential fatty acids, and vitamin D, or using targeted therapies such as SAMe, cranial electrical stimulation, and bright light therapy, options for intervention multiply. Consideration of health and wellness parameters such as education around a whole food diet and minimization of environmental toxic exposures supports a healthy pregnancy and postpartum experience for mother and baby.

REFERENCES

1. Heron J, O'Connor TG, Evans J, et al. The course of anxiety and depression through pregnancy and the postpartum in a community sample. J Affect Disord 2004;80(1):65–73.
2. Lorenzo L, Byers B, Einarson A. Antidepressant use in pregnancy. Expert Opin Drug Saf 2011;10(6):883–9.
3. Freeman MP. Complementary and alternative medicine for perinatal depression. J Affect Disord 2009;112(1–3):1–10.
4. Cerutti R, Sichel MP, Perin M, et al. Psychological distress during puerperium: a novel therapeutic approach using S-adenosylmethionine. Curr Ther Res 1993;53:707–16.
5. Gunther M, Phillips K. Cranial electrotherapy stimulation for the treatment of depression. Journal of Psychosocial Nursing 2010;1–6.
6. Hibbeln JR. Seafood consumption, the DHA content of mothers' milk and prevalence rates of postpartum depression: a cross-national, ecological analysis. J Affect Disord 2002;69(1–3):15–29.
7. Strøm M, Mortensen EL, Halldorsson TI, et al. Fish and long-chain n-3 polyunsaturated fatty acid intakes during pregnancy and risk of postpartum depression: a prospective study based on a large national birth cohort. Am J Clin Nutr 2009;90(1):149–55.
8. Lin PY, Su KP. A meta-analytic review of double-blind, placebo-controlled trials of antidepressant efficacy of omega-3 fatty acids. J Clin Psychiatry 2007;68(7):1056–61.
9. Sublette ME, Ellis SP, Geant AL, et al. Meta-analysis of the effects of eicosapentaenoic acid (EPA) in clinical trials in depression. J Clin Psychiatry 2011;10032:1–8.
10. Niculescu MD, Lupu DS, Craciunescu CN. Perinatal manipulation of α-linolenic acid intake induces epigenetic changes in maternal and offspring livers. FASEB J 2012;1:1–9.
11. Rubin D, Laposata M. Cellular interactions between n-6 and n-3 fatty acids: a mass analysis of fatty acid elongation/desaturation, distribution among complex lipids, and conversion to eicosanoids. J Lipid Res 1992;33(10):1431–40.
12. Horrobin DF, Bennett CN. New gene targets related to schizophrenia and other psychiatric disorders: enzymes, binding proteins and transport proteins involved in phospholipid and fatty acid metabolism. Prostaglandins Leukot Essent Fatty Acids 1999;60(3):141–67.
13. Horrobin D. The role of essential fatty acids and prostaglandins in the premenstrual syndrome. J Reprod Med 1983;28:465–8.

14. Geppert J, Demmelmair H, Hornstra G, et al. Co-supplementation of healthy women with fish oil and evening primrose oil increases plasma docosahexaenoic acid, gamma-linolenic acid and dihomo-gamma-linolenic acid levels without reducing arachidonic acid concentrations. Br J Nutr 2008;99(2):360–9.
15. Devlin AM, Brain U, Austin J, et al. Prenatal exposure to maternal depressed mood and the MTHFR C677T variant affect SLC6A4 methylation in infants at birth. PloS One 2010;5(8):e12201.
16. Lewis SJ, Araya R, Leary S, et al. Folic acid supplementation during pregnancy may protect against depression 21 months after pregnancy, an effect modified by MTHFR C677T genotype. Eur J Clin Nutr 2011;1–7.
17. Cassidy-Bushrow AE, Peters RM, Johnson DA, et al. Vitamin D nutritional status and antenatal depressive symptoms in African American women. J Womens Health (Larchmt) 2012;21(11):1189–95.
18. Wagner CL, Taylor SN, Johnson DD, et al. The role of vitamin D in pregnancy and lactation: emerging concepts. Womens Health 2012;8(3):323–40.
19. Brandenbarg J, Vrijkotte TG, Goedhart G, et al. Maternal early-pregnancy vitamin D status is associated with maternal depressive symptoms in the Amsterdam born children and their development cohort. Psychosom Med 2012;1–7.
20. Murphy PK, Mueller M, Hulsey TC, et al. An exploratory study of postpartum depression and vitamin D. J Am Psychiatr Nurses Assoc 2010;16(3):170–7.
21. Giddens JB, Krug SK, Tsang RS, et al. Pregnant adolescent and adult women have similarly low intakes of selected nutrients. J Am Diet Assoc 2000;100(11):1334–40.
22. Sylvén SM, Elenis E, Michelakos T, et al. Thyroid function tests at delivery and risk for postpartum depressive symptoms. Psychoneuroendocrinology 2012. [Epub ahead of print].
23. Bergink V, Kushner SA, Pop V, et al. Prevalence of autoimmune thyroid dysfunction in postpartum psychosis. Br J Psychiatry 2011;198(4):264–8.
24. Cooke R, Russell J, Levitt A. T3 augmentation of antidepressant treatment in T4-replaced thyroid patients. J Clin Psychiatry 1992;16–8.
25. Corwin EJ, Johnston N, Pugh L. Symptoms of postpartum depression associated with elevated levels of interleukin-1 beta during the first month postpartum. Biol Res Nurs 2008;10(2):128–33.
26. Lindstrom L, Nyberg F, Terenius L. CSF and plasma B-casomorphin-like opioid peptides in postpartum psychosis. Am J Psychiatry 1984;141(9):1059–66.
27. Karlsson H, Wicks S. Maternal antibodies to dietary antigens and risk for nonaffective psychosis in offspring. Am J Psychiatry 2012;1–8.
28. Jurewicz J, Hanke W. Exposure to phthalates: reproductive outcome and children health. A review of epidemiological studies. Int J Occup Med Environ Health 2011;24(2):115–41.
29. Gascon M, Vrijheid M, Martínez D, et al. Effects of pre and postnatal exposure to low levels of polybromodiphenyl ethers on neurodevelopment and thyroid hormone levels at 4years of age. Environ Int 2011;37(3):605–11.
30. Braun JM, Kalkbrenner AE, Calafat AM, et al. Impact of early-life bisphenol A exposure on behavior and executive function in children. Pediatrics 2011;128:873–82.

Index

Note: Page numbers of article titles are in **boldface** type.

Psychiatr Clin N Am 36 (2013) 189–199
http://dx.doi.org/10.1016/S0193-953X(13)00020-8
0193-953X/13/$ – see front matter © 2013 Elsevier Inc. All rights reserved.